THIS IS

Motor Boating

Other titles in this series

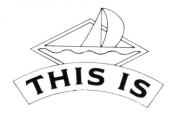

THIS IS
Motor Boating

Ramon Gliewe

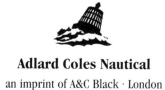

Adlard Coles Nautical

an imprint of A&C Black · London

First edition 1992
Published by Adlard Coles Nautical
an imprint of
A & C Black (Publishers) Ltd
35 Bedford Row, London WC1R 4JH

© United Nautical Publishers SA, Basel, Switzerland, 1992

ISBN 0 7136 3458 8

A CIP catalogue record for this book is available from the
British Library.

Typeset in Times New Roman by August Filmsetting, St Helens.
Printed and bound in Italy

Contents

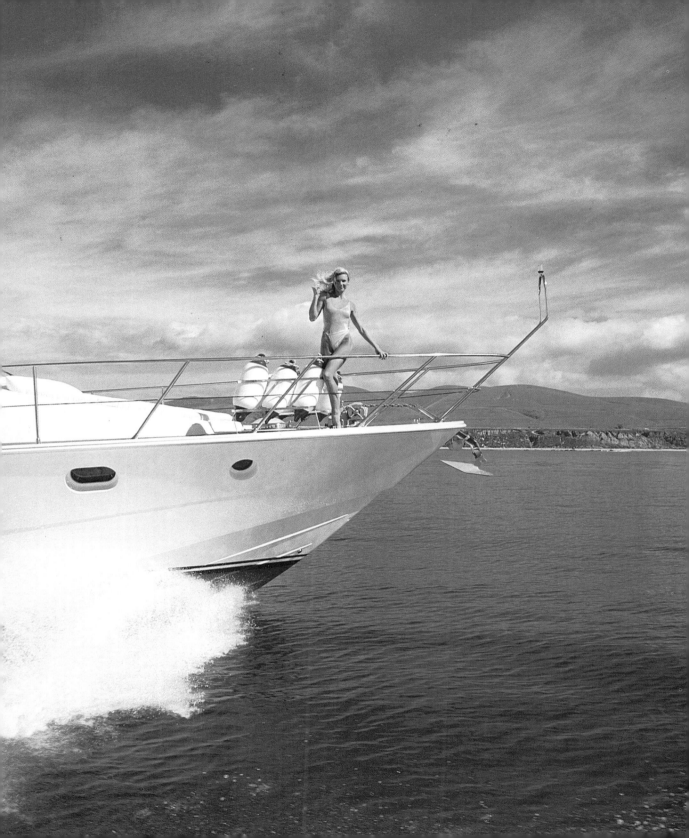

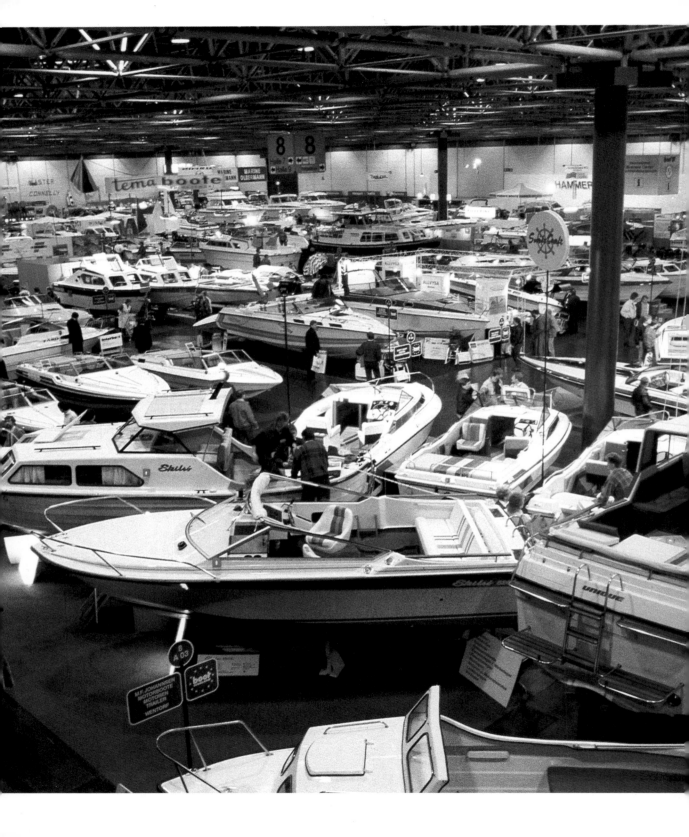

Which boat for what purpose?

If the first thing you want to know is 'the price', a boat show exhibitor replied to a questioner, 'our yachts are not for you anyway'. Fair enough, maybe, since those prices were around a quarter of a million pounds. However, the great majority of motorboaters unfortunately do have to reconcile their wishes and dreams somehow with the state of their bank balance.

You have to look beyond the purchase price of the boat. The first extra is the additional essential equipment – usually not included in the price. Then the running costs, just for fuel and maintenance, amount to a great deal more than they do with cars. Also, you have to take into account the cost of the summer berth and the winter quarters. So the chief question isn't: 'How much does the boat cost?', but rather 'How much can I afford to spend on my boat annually?'

Leaving the financial constraints aside altogether, there is the problem of finding the 'right' boat for one's particular purposes. It is a fact that very many people, having decided to take to the water, have considerable difficulty in forming a picture of the qualities desirable in their boat and of its power requirements. The choice is just too overwhelmingly large; the range of shapes and types are too confusing. Let us try to bring some order into this confusion.

Motor boats can be classified according to certain constructional characteristics or type of power unit.

An International Boat Show is a good place to look and compare, but you should never buy a boat without having a trial run first.

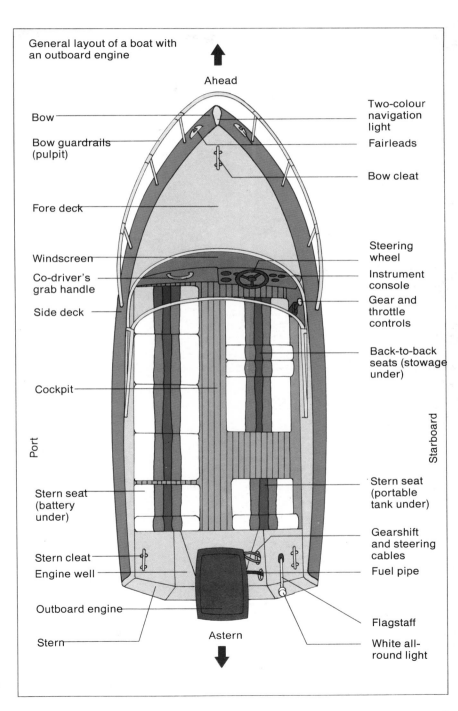

General layout of a boat with an outboard engine

Ahead

Bow

Bow guardrails (pulpit)

Fore deck

Windscreen

Co-driver's grab handle

Side deck

Cockpit

Port

Stern seat (battery under)

Stern cleat

Engine well

Outboard engine

Stern

Two-colour navigation light

Fairleads

Bow cleat

Steering wheel

Instrument console

Gear and throttle controls

Back-to-back seats (stowage under)

Starboard

Stern seat (portable tank under)

Gearshift and steering cables

Fuel pipe

Flagstaff

White all-round light

Astern

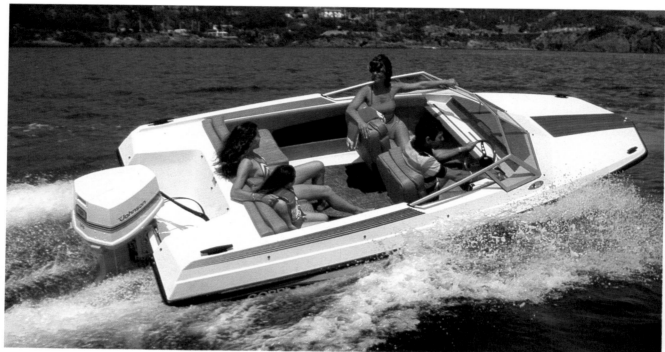

This is a popular type of GRP sports boat with a powerful outboard. This boat has seats for the driver and co-driver, and a full-width stern bench for four people.

Even the smallest rowing dinghy turns into a motor boat if you hang one of those egg-whisk outboards over its stern, but such baby boats with auxiliary power we shall exclude from our considerations. Let us first look around the lower end of the range, at the open-cockpit boat probably typical of what most motorboaters own: the open outboard powered sports boat, length 4 metres and upwards. It usually has a foredeck and four upholstered seats in the cockpit. In the more comfortable versions these seats are arranged back-to-

back and can be extended to form sunbeds. For the young, even camping on board for the odd night with a tarpaulin over the cockpit is possible. There are often small stowage recesses along the sides and at the stern.

These are fast boats, to be driven sportingly; up to about 5 or 6 metres long, with engines ranging from 20 hp (15 kW)* up to 100 hp (73 kW) depending on size. Such high-powered craft are of course not for beginners, their proper control calls for highly

*According to the international units system SI, hp ceased to exist after 1.1.1978. The power unit for engines valid since then is the kilowatt (kW). However the engine builders have so far been unable to agree a standard kW-rating and the motorboaters are reluctant to abandon the familiar hp. Accordingly, hp will also be used predominantly here.

developed driving skills. This type of boat permits extensive outings in sheltered waters and has the space for the bits and pieces four people need for a day. This size of boat competes with the sports-inflatable of 4–5 metre length, powered by outboard engines up to about 75 hp (55 kW). Mind you, from a price point of view, the inflatable is scarcely competitive: with the same equipment, it costs about 35% more than a same-size rigid boat. This extra cost arises from the complications involved in the manufacture and assembly of their hulls. But – and here the comparison becomes interesting – inflatables are about 45% lighter than rigid boats of corresponding size. That means that they can make do with a substantially less powerful engine for the same speed, which recoups some of the higher purchase

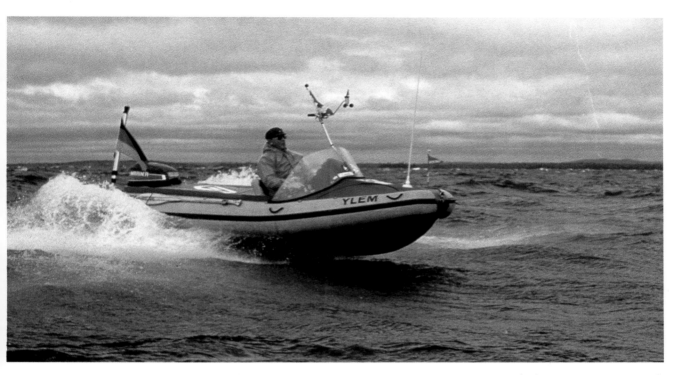

This 4 metre sports inflatable has a rigid hull and will handle remarkably well in choppy water. Note the cockpit cover to stop spray or breaking seas from filling the boat.

price of the hull. It also means less fuel for the same speed, which in turn reduces the operating costs.

But the most important argument in the inflatable's favour lies in the safety of their inherent buoyancy. A fully laden two-chamber boat – there are several models with even more chambers – will continue to float even with only one air chamber intact, and remains driveable and manoeuvrable to some extent even if the cockpit is submerged. It is practically unsinkable and in that respect is superior to comparable rigid boats.

It is this quality which time and again encourages drivers of inflatables to undertake extensive open sea cruises: runs across the Aegean, around the Balearics and the Canaries and even across the Med, to Tunisia and Egypt. Such trips are entirely

practicable provided plans and preparations have been made thoroughly and they are undertaken by a crew experienced in navigation and the ways of the sea. One thing is certain though, these 'pocket boats', whether inflatable or rigid, are not intended for open sea work. They are designed for sheltered waters, for river trips, for fair weather runs within sight of the coast. That point must not be obscured even by the speed they can attain if powerfully engined, which enables them to cover a lot of ground in a short time. The same reservations also apply to open sports boats with inboard engines, sometimes referred to as runabouts. Their typical length ranges between 5 and 8 metres and power units are usually inboard engines up to about 170 hp (125 kW). As well as the four back-to-back seats

they usually have two more seats at the stern alongside the engine casing, but their interior scarcely differs from that of the elegant outboard craft. Some dispense with the deck over the forebody in favour of a forward cockpit. Separated from the main cockpit by the fascia and the windscreen and anyway not usable at high speed, it is a feature of somewhat dubious value.

In the range of overlap between outboard and inboard engined boats, both types of power unit are often on offer for one and the same hull. If you'd like to go a bit faster you could choose the outboard version, because an outboard engine is about 50% lighter for much the same power output and so the boat's maximum speed goes up by a few knots. A point overlooked all too often when considering the engine for a boat is that the more powerful engine is usually heavier and swallows up a part of its power gain for its own (increased) weight. The heavier same-power inboard engine in the slower boat, however, is generally less thirsty than the other. But if you pick a proportionately less powerful outboard which will nevertheless give you substantially the same maximum speed, the fuel consumption balance again works out in favour of the outboard. The larger inboard-engined types obviously offer more by way of comfort, larger stowage spaces and more comprehensive engine instrumentation.

If you're aiming a little higher, you end up with the day-cruiser type of sportsboat: boats up to about 8 metres in length, single- or twin-engined up to 225 hp (166 kW). Often without a raised cabin structure, they can have elegant lines and a racy low profile. However appearances may be deceptive; they're cabin boats but the cabin has been integrated into the foredeck. It usually houses only small lockers and two bunks; sometimes also a cooking-area and foodstore. Inevitably, there cannot be much space or headroom and the accommodation provides its comforts on a miniature scale.

This kind of sportsboat is primarily

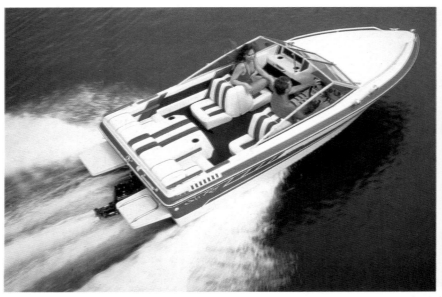

This sports boat has an inboard engine and room for six people, with two extendable back-to-back seats and two more alongside the engine casing which is also upholstered. When planing at high speed, the aft seats are the most comfortable; the hull hits the waves near the driver's position.

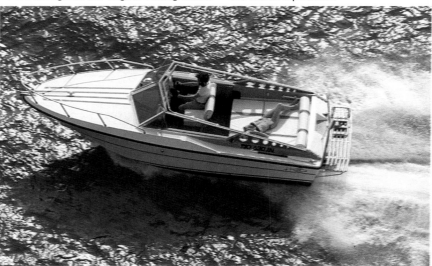

This day cruiser has basic overnight facilities with a cabin below the foredeck. The extensive sun deck on top of the engine casing is a typical feature; it provides two improvised sleeping berths under a cockpit awning. A full width bathing platform at the stern also protects the outdrive.

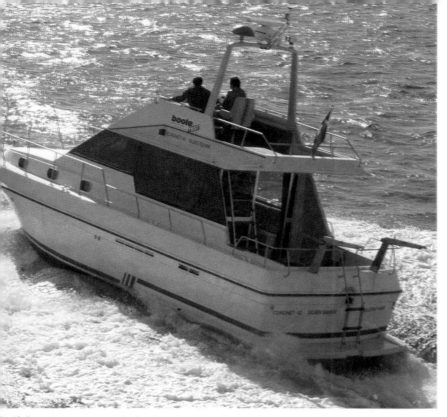

A 12.5 metre motor yacht for fast, comfortable cruising. This type of boat usually has twin engines driving fixed shafts.
Typical is the flybridge with the second
helming position above a deck level
saloon, which houses the main helming
position.

designed for day trips and occasional
weekend cruising. This doesn't mean,
at least with the larger versions, that
you can't also undertake longer passages involving open sea crossings.
They are seaworthy up to a certain
point and skippers always have to
take careful account of the weather.
What makes the day-cruiser so
interesting for many people is the ease
of moving it by land. Its weight is low
enough for it to be towed on a trailer
without difficulty and it can be driven
to wherever the boating conditions are
most pleasant.

Related to the day-cruiser are the
half-cabin boats with a sort of open-
at-the-back hardtop usually extend-
ing over the helming position; at one
time they were very popular, but lately
they have gone out of fashion somewhat. Beneath the hardtop there are

bunks and a simple galley. By cover-
ing it with a reinforced awning the
cockpit may be partially included in
the 'living space'. It was – and still is –
typically a boat for the young.

If you decide to buy a more comfortable boat with a cabin, then this
often means the end of delivery trips
by land because the boat is too heavy
to be towed on a trailer by car. You
will need a permanent berth as a base
for all outings; in return you get
enough height to stand upright on
board and the comfort of at least one
spacious cabin. Sometimes there's an
after cabin as well. There will be several adequately sized bunks, a dining
area, a galley with a multi-burner
cooker and running water, and separate toilet, sometimes with a shower.
Frequently, there is a steering position
in the cabin so that the helmsman is

not continually exposed to the rigours
of wind, rain or spray.

This category comprises boats
ranging in length from about 8 to 12
metres. Within this range the level of
accommodation and comfort varies
widely, and so the number of berths
and separate cabins available. The
title 'cruiser' or 'motor-cruiser', usual
in the past for cabin boats from about
8 metres upwards, is now no longer
used so much, but it describes their
potential pretty well. These are boats
for lengthier voyages, with sufficient
stowage space for the stores needed,
lockers for personal belongings, and
larger tanks for drinking water and
fuel. Such cabin boats may be fitted
with one or two inboard engines,
which are usually diesel.

The larger cruisers are often equipped with a second helming position up
on the coach roof, the so-called flybridge. With its comfortably upholstered sofa benches, the flybridge can
serve as a small sundeck. Up there,
you can enjoy the sea air and – the
most important feature – have a better
all-round view when manoeuvring.

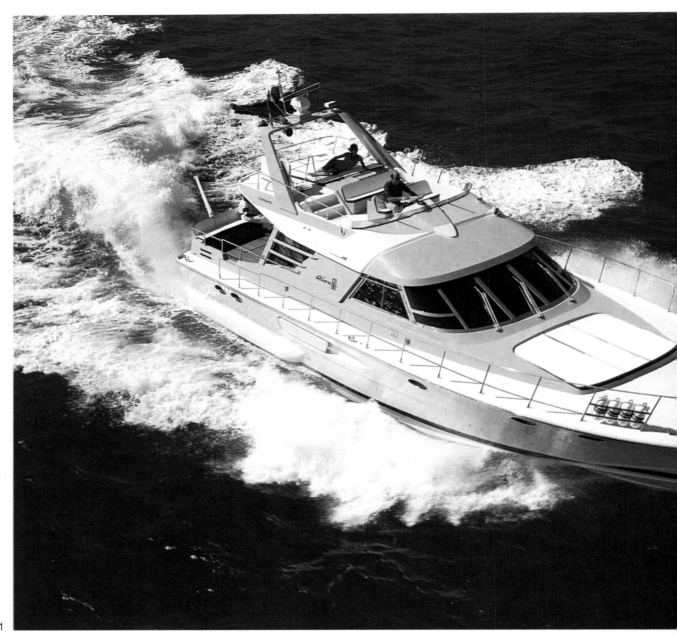

1

A dream of luxury and sparkling performance, and all in barely 17 metres:

1 *Corsaro*, a fine example of the Italian boat builder's art. The Italians are currently the leading designers of large, comfortable and fast motor yachts. The full throated roar of 2×760 hp MAN diesels brings this 40-tonner up to a maximum speed of 30 knots. At a cruising speed of 26 knots she can cover 400 miles, and be under way for 15 hours without refuelling. The flybridge is on two

levels; right aft there is a large sun deck and in front of this, two steps lower, is the helming position with two two-seater benches.

2 A row of ceiling lights provides generous illumination for the saloon in the deckhouse with its lounge and dining areas. Protected by the large panoramic screen, the comfortable helming position is equipped with radar, marine radio, and 'domestic' intercom. Alongside this, a companionway leads down to

the lower compartments including the galley. A sea water desalination plant can produce 1200 litres of fresh water daily to fill the 700 litre tanks.

3 A look into the 'bedroom' of another Italian dream yacht. The 18.3 metre 48-ton Sealine 18 is also powered by two 760 hp MAN diesels. She has a maximum speed of 32 knots and even at cruising speed still cuts a dash at 28 knots. The sophisticated modern furniture and fittings might almost be enough to make

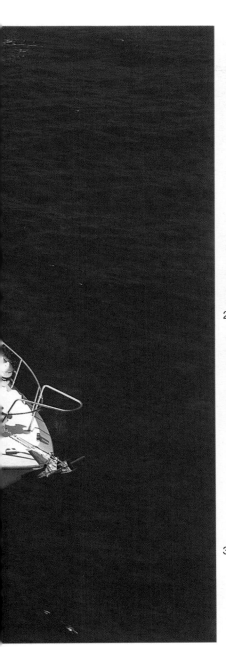

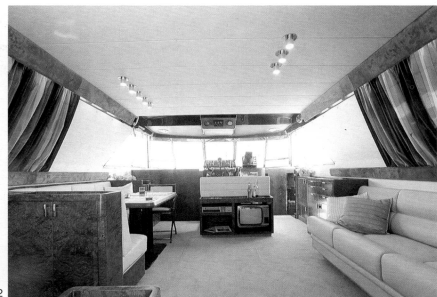

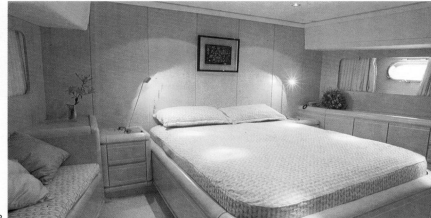

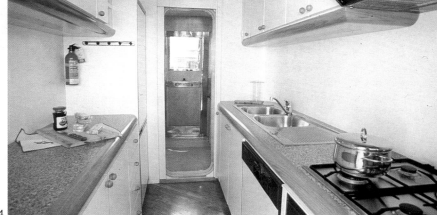

you forget that you are at sea.

4   In the Sealine's galley, it is a pleasure to cook for yourself and your guests. From a fume extractor hood above the four burner cooker with oven, through to an electric grill, to a chest deep freeze, there is no need to do without any of your creature comforts.

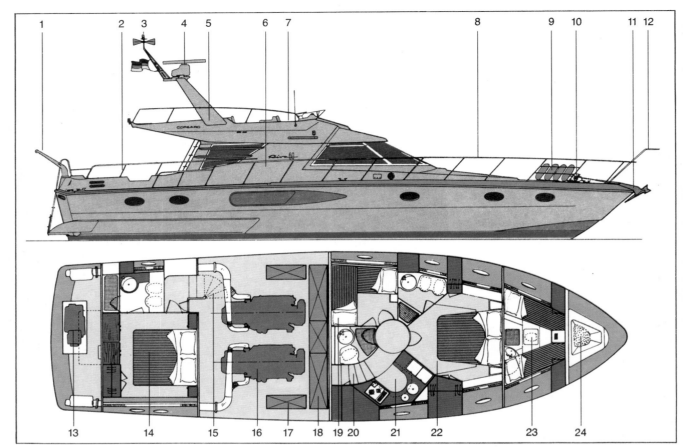

Profile and internal plan of an 18.7 metre luxury yacht, whose twin 760 hp engines give a maximum speed of 30 knots.

1 Davit
2 Cockpit with access to flybridge
3 Steaming light
4 Radar
5 Flying gantry for radar scanner, aerials etc
6 Deck-level saloon with lounge and dining areas and the main helming position
7 Flybridge with outer helming position
8 Guardrails
9 Fender stowage
10 Anchor winch
11 Anchor ready for letting go
12 Pulpit
13 Generator
14 Owner's cabin with double bed and toilet with shower
15 Way down to machinery space
16 Twin-engine installation
17 Fresh water tanks
18 Fuel tanks
19 Guest cabin with single beds tiered to form an 'L', and toilet with shower
20 Way down to fore part
21 Galley
22 Second owner's cabin or large guest cabin with double bed and toilet with shower
23 Crew's quarters with two bunks, heads and basin. Access via fore-hatch
24 Cable locker

A few special designs and fancy craft apart, most boats up to motor cruiser size are built of GRP. For larger motor cruisers, though, other materials besides GRP are also used: solid wood (though this is rare) moulded plywood, steel or aluminium.

And now we have reached that class of boat whose purchasers don't enquire too closely about the price – the motor yachts. These vessels are of some 13 metres or more in length –

there isn't really an upper limit. They accommodate, often spread over several deck levels, sleeping cabins and bathrooms fitted out from pretty comfortable to luxurious. There will usually be owner's, guests', and crew cabins.

Nothing is missing, from microwave oven to video and radio equipment, so that you feel on board as though you were at home and the ultra modern engine technology and

navigational electronics are similar to those on a cruise liner. On this type of yacht, instead of referring to a helming position you had better call it a bridge. Engines of 2500 hp (1800 kW) or more draw their fuel from 6000 litre capacity tanks.

These are fully seaworthy, powerful yachts for lengthy voyages. If they are more than 60–70 metres long, you might see a helicopter-pad on deck as well as a swimming pool.

Planing or displacement craft – what do these terms mean?

Motor boats up to day cruiser size are often straightforward planing craft; of the smaller motor cruisers some are and some aren't. That doesn't mean that there are no day cruiser size boats conceived as displacement craft by their designer. And that pitches us into the middle of a sort of philosophical divide between motor boaters: planers on one side, displacers on the other. 'Which type of hull is most suitable for the type of boating I want to do?' Displacement boats have become much less popular in the last few years, but are now starting to come back into favour.

Planing craft have their advantages and limitations. There's a rule of thumb which says that only boats weighing less than 16 kg per hp (22 kg per kW) can plane properly. So planing craft must either weigh very little – a condition no longer fulfilled in the cases of larger boats – or they must have very powerful engines. As a consequence, fast they may be, but economical they certainly are not. A displacement craft, on the other hand, can get away with a minimum of power; it travels relatively slowly and extremely economically. Here, various hydrodynamic and hydrostatic factors are at work, which significantly influence everything that happens at the hull surface of a boat under way. It was the Greek mathematician and physicist Archimedes who discovered that a body floating in water displaces its own weight. Now 1 m³ of water weighs about a tonne; so if the volume of a body weighing 1 tonne

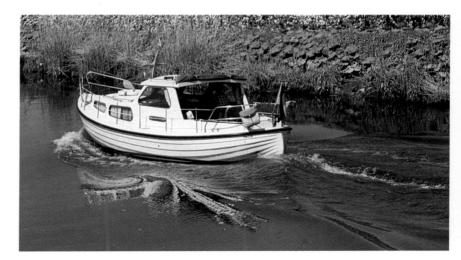

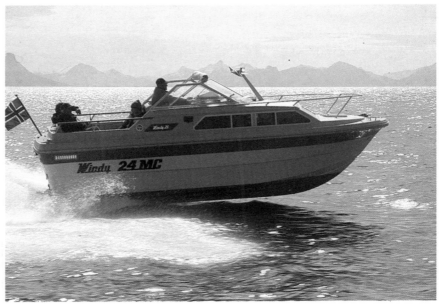

Displacement or planing craft
Two different outlooks on life – the displacement craft, slow but economical; the planing craft, sporting, cutting a dash, but very thirsty. The two illustrations clearly show the differences in behaviour under way of two boats of the same size. The displacement craft sits between its bow and stern wave – it can't get away from these. The wave pattern shows that the boat is already running at her limiting speed; she can go no faster. The planing craft rises above its bow wave, the forebody is clear of the water and only the aft third is riding on the 'bow wave'. The boat is running at the ideal planing speed and could make a few more knots.

exceeds 1 m³, it will submerge only far enough to displace 1 m³ of water. That is the whole secret of why even ships made of iron float. For this reason also, the weight of yachts is sometimes given in m³ of displacement. Figuratively speaking, a boat at rest lies in a trough in the water created by its own weight. As soon as the boat starts moving it has to take that trough with it, push it along underneath its belly as it were. As a result of this progress, bow and stern waves are generated at the water surface. The mass of water pushed aside, ie displaced, always corresponds to the boat's weight. If you keep that in mind, you will understand why there is a limit to the speed a heavy boat can achieve, for as the speed increases so does the displacement effort. The resistance offered by the water to the hull ploughing through it increases as the square of the speed, until finally all that happens is that a system of high waves is generated in which the boat remains inescapably embedded. Beyond a certain point, the only use the boat can make of additional engine power is to dig itself a deeper trough in the water and throw up higher waves at bow and stern. At the same time, the frictional resistance on the submerged surface also increases all the time and holds on to the boat.

Planing craft behave quite differently. That same water resistance which impedes high speed in the displacement craft, the planing craft uses to increase its speed. Its underside forms an attack surface for the water. As the speed increases, this lifts the boat further out of the water so that ultimately it is merely skidding over the surface. Put another way, planing craft work their way out of their displacement trough, push themselves up

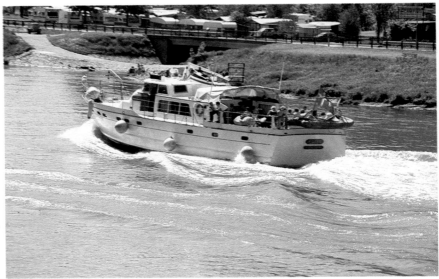

A wave pattern typical of larger vessels. This displacement craft is running at between a third and a half of its limiting speed. You can see the first hull wave just forward of midships. As the speed increases towards the limiting speed, this wave will move aft to become the stern wave.

on to their bow wave and leave their stern wave far behind. The further that drops astern, the higher the planing speed. What makes this possible is a so-called dynamic buoyancy underneath the hull which supports the bow and part of the forebody. A boat when planing thus becomes 'lighter', ie it displaces less water than its weight equivalent. For that reason it produces only a slight wash. The wetted area of the hull and thus the frictional resistance is substantially reduced. But the generation of that dynamic buoyancy in the first instance calls for a powerful engine: until the boat attains planing speed, it is behaving in the same way as a displacement craft.

The secrets of relative speed

Immediately a mass of questions arises, with which the motorboater finds himself confronted time and again: is there any possibility of assessing whether a boat is really capable of the speed which the builder claims for it? When is a boat fully planing? When is it running economically? Does more horsepower mean better seakeeping qualities? What is meant by the hull- or limiting speed, which displacement craft reputedly can't exceed and sometimes don't even attain? It was the English physicist William Froude who, in 1872, managed to penetrate the secret of the waves.

He discovered a law connecting the length of a wave – from crest to crest – with the speed of advance of the wave trains. Equal speeds of advance also always mean equal wave lengths. Conversely, you can deduce speed of advance from wave length. Any ship under way, by pushing water aside, produces a system of waves. These waves advance at the same speed as the ship through the water, no matter how large or heavy the ship. This discovery of Froude's led to the formula for 'relative speed' – R, or sometimes written V_R. It is calculated as follows:

$$R = \frac{\text{boat's speed in kph or knots}}{\sqrt{\text{waterline length in metres}}}$$

This relative speed is the key to understanding the connection between hull shape, speed and engine power. It makes possible a speed comparison between boats of different sizes and indicates whether a certain type of hull will measure up to the salesman's promises. It demonstrates whether design and engine power match. The importance of relative speed can be demonstrated by an example. A 4 metre boat capable of 20 km/h we would consider as fast, but a 20 km/h 15 metre yacht would look pretty tame. That impression does not deceive, for the relative speeds compare as follows:

$$4\,\text{m boat: } \frac{20}{2} = 10$$

$$15\,\text{m yacht: } \frac{20}{3.87} = 5.2$$

The absolute speed at 20 km/h is identical, but the little 4 metre boat with R = 10 is relatively twice as fast as the large yacht with R = 5.2.

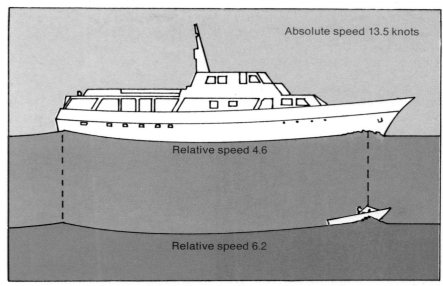

Absolute speed 13.5 knots

Relative speed 4.6

Relative speed 6.2

Amazing but true: at the same absolute speed, every vessel, be it an inflatable dinghy or a super tanker, makes waves of the same length. However the 30 metre yacht (in our example) cruising at displacement speed nestles between her bow and stern wave. The 6 metre boat travelling at the same speed is planing on its bow wave but has left its stern wave far behind.

R = 4.5 (speed in km/h) or R = 2.43 (speed in knots) is the theoretical hull- or limiting speed which displacement craft normally can't exceed. The wave length then is exactly the same as the waterline length of the hull in question. But whether a displacement craft can actually attain its hull speed or whether perhaps the engine lacks the necessary power can easily be calculated if you know the waterline length (WL):

$\sqrt{\text{WL(m)}} \times 4.5 = \text{hull speed in km/h}$;
$\sqrt{\text{WL(m)}} \times 2.43 = \text{hull speed in knots}$ (nautical miles per hour).

(For simplicity's sake we shall from now on do calculations in km/h only.)

A displacement craft has the advantage that it requires only a relatively modest amount of power (6 hp/ 4.5 kW per tonne) to attain its maximum speed. Its economy, particularly if driven by a diesel, is thus one of the principal points in its favour. Installing more powerful and therefore more expensive and thirstier engines than required is self-defeating. You simply generate a deep wave trough and a high stern wave to which the stern remains glued. Beyond R = 4.5, doubling the engine power of a classic displacement craft produces only about 10% more speed.

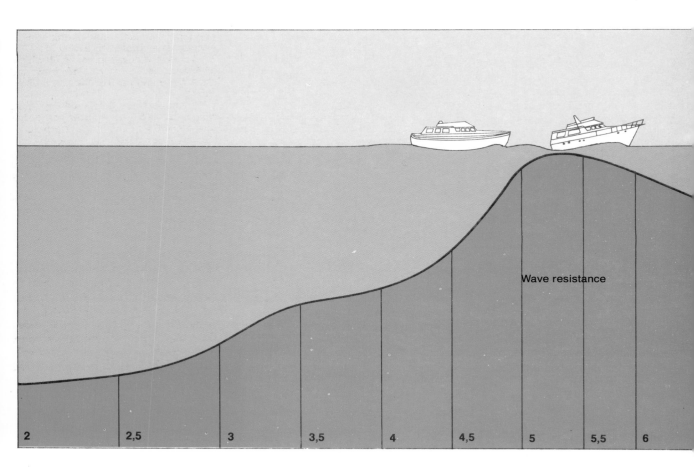

Wave resistance

| 2 | 2,5 | 3 | 3,5 | 4 | 4,5 | 5 | 5,5 | 6 |

A displacement boat traditionally has a round-bilge hull with a keel of varying depth and a rounded stern. This type of hull is generally considered particularly seaworthy. By virtue of their keel, boats built like this are pretty stable directionally and behave predictably in rough seas; although they are inclined to roll uncomfortably in beam seas. Sometimes the contemplative speed of travel of displacement craft, so beloved of their devotees, can become a handicap on river journeys if you

have difficulty avoiding commercial traffic or breasting a strong current. Nevertheless, anyone who intends predominantly to sail in waters where speed limits apply – for example many of the European inland waterways and canals – can safely opt for a displacement boat. Its hull shape is ideal for leisurely travel. Planing craft are extremely skittish on the rudder when going slowly, and dawdling doesn't really suit their powerful engines either.

Fast displacement craft

However, there *are* displacement craft capable of exceeding their theoretical hull speed. This is usually achieved by means of a constructional trick, perhaps by having a wide transom or cutaway stern, and by using more power. Such boats can rise to a relative speed R = 5.5 and people tend to call them fast or even 'superfast' displacement craft. There is, of course, no longer much of a connection with

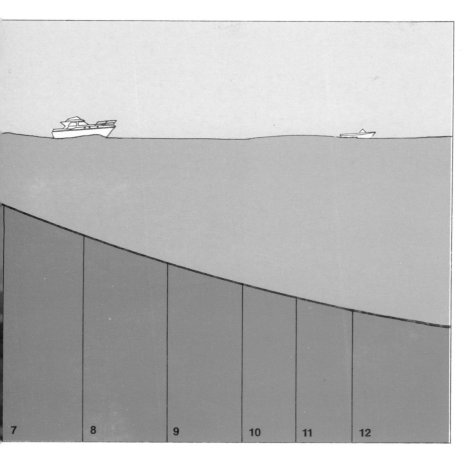

The high resistance hump which gives every boat a problem to overcome:
1   A classical displacement craft which, at R=4.5, is hemmed-in by bow and stern wave and has reached its limiting speed.
2   A 'superfast' displacement craft which, at R=5.5, is right on top of the resistance hump and has its stern hanging down into a deep wave trough.
3   The semi-displacement craft which, at R=8, has left the resistance hump behind and is running substantially flatter.
4   The planing craft at R=12 or more is running nearly flat and makes only minimal waves.

Instead of ploughing on at full power, it is substantially more economical to reduce speed to less than R=5. Or, even better, to install less horsepower in the first place. Anyone who cares about fuel consumption should avoid boats which, at full power, just reach the high resistance hump with R values between 5 and 7.

Semi-displacement craft

A true transition between displacement and planing craft is the genuine semi-displacement craft, sometimes called an express cruiser. The underwater hull has a planing form, but is too heavy to be brought up to planing speed by the engine fitted. These craft, usually motor cruisers, have a weight/power ratio between 16 and 30 kg/hp (22 and 41 kg/kW). Since there is a considerable build up of dynamic pressure under the hull, which lifts the boat out of the water to some extent and thus reduces frictional resistance and displacement, the 'R' values of a semi-displacement boat typically lie between 8 and 10. If

economical running. Even with the most favourably shaped stern, a mighty stern wave is built up and fuel consumption is heavy. When R=5.25, every vessel is sailing in the zone of maximum wave resistance. The so-called resistance hump which arises here is a natural phenomenon and not to be easily outwitted by any constructional tricks. The especially pronounced wave formation can be splendidly observed on any vessel travelling in that speed range. Naturally, planing craft must pass through

this speed range as they accelerate – they are also running uneconomically and with a high stern wave when R=5.25.

Just like the true displacement craft, a fast displacement boat remains trapped in its wave, only it no longer builds up at the end of its waterline – since this has in a manner of speaking been cut back – but rather a bit astern of the transom. Such boats frequently cause an unpleasant wash. Many large motor yachts classified as displacement craft belong in this category.

Planing craft attitudes:
1 R = 4. Slow running in displacement mode. Attitude horizontal. Little wave generation. Relatively low fuel consumption.
2 R = 5.25. On the resistance hump. Stern sagging, bow up in the air. The most uneconomical operating speed. To get away from this, the boat needs a lot of power. So don't increase the revs gradually – that means spending more time stuck in this uneconomical transition phase; give it all you've got straightaway.
3 R = 8. Dynamic lift raises the stern; the nose comes down. Planing starts. (Economical speed for semi-displacement craft.)
4 R-12 (and more). Proper planing. Hull angle of incidence about 2°. Minimal wave generation.

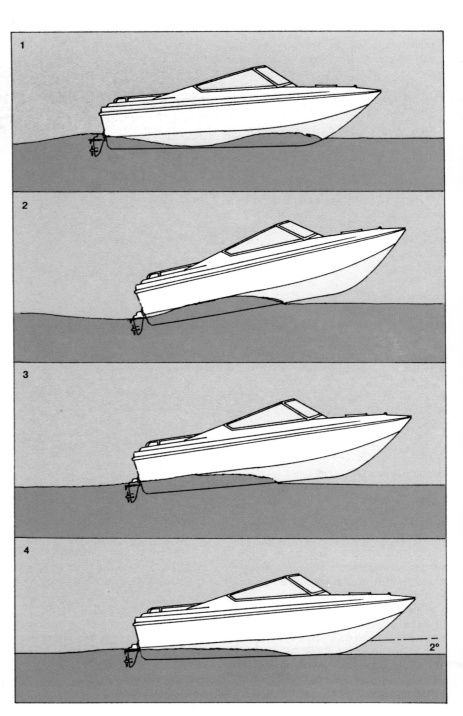

this relative speed isn't achieved, either the hull has design faults or the engine is too feeble.

Although semi-displacement boats operate out of the unfavourable resistance zone and wave formation is much reduced, they sometimes trim badly, which in turn swallows up power. The cause of this is the combination of two forces: dynamic lift for the relatively light bows and static sag for a stern made excessively heavy by powerful engines. Sometimes you see boats of this kind tearing along nose-in-the-air, which can be even less economical than a fast displacement craft. Some correction is possible by means of trim tabs. In reality, all fast motor cruisers longer than about 10–11 metres are designed as semi-displacement craft. For very large boats, longer than about 17–18 metres, displacement hulls are the norm, largely on weight and power grounds.

There are exceptions though. If you think it's worth the money to install

3000 hp engines, fit special racing gearboxes and props and burn 200 gallons of fuel every hour, you can get your 21 metre boat (17 metre WL) to do a full 100 km/h. With R = 24.2, this would undeniably be planing. The Italians specialize in fast super yachts for owners who really don't have to ask about the price. Proper planing for recreational boating normally occurs in the R = 12 to (perhaps) R = 30 range, depending on weight, hull shape and engine power of the boat. Anything above that belongs unquestionably in the racer category. R = 30, for instance in the case of a 6 metre waterline length boat, amounts to 73 km/h ($\sqrt{6 \times 30}$) – and that's quite a speed. Intoxication, to skim over a mirrorlike surface that fast. But water is rarely like that, a sad fact which, among their opponents, has earned planing and semi-displacement craft the reputation of rough riders. Because what the protagonists of planing still describe as 'soft immersion', the displacement man considers to be hard slamming.

What planing craft underwater hulls reveal

To some extent, you can judge from the look of a planing craft's underwater hull what performance to expect in choppy water. If you haven't understood the meaning of 'deep V' before, you will appreciate it now. In boat brochures and test reports you might read about the deadrise angle of the bottom. In the case of a true deep V, this lies between 22° and 26°, all the way from stem to stern. Such boats ride relatively softly but need more (at least 10% more) horsepower to reach

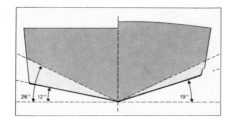

Hull underside shapes. Deep 'V' with 26° deadrise (broken line) all the way from stem to stern. Nowadays little used for recreational craft. Modern modified 'V' with 12° deadrise over the after two thirds (left) and 19° over the forward third.

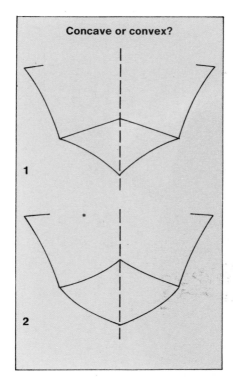

1 Typical forward lines of earlier planing craft with concave bottom sections and relatively low straight chine.
2 Modern forebody with convex bottom sections and the chine curved and rising towards the bow.

the same speed as a flatter-V hull – understandably, since the immersed (wetted) surface is greater than with a flatter bottom and thus more frictional resistance has to be overcome. Boats at the upper weight limit of 15 kg/hp (20 kg/kW) may well be impossible to plane without trim tabs.

Undersides which have the portion flatter by 10° to 15° are a good compromise. Today's successful planing designs have undersides with a deadrise of about 12° over the after two-thirds of the hull, and up to 19° in the forward third merging with slightly outward-curving (convex) sections near the bows. The chine – the pronounced kink along both sides – has to be drawn upwards strongly towards the bows so that it can fling the spray sideways. If the part of the forebody below that kink is concave (inward-curving) it's a certainty that the boat will slam into even the smallest wave and the only place where there's a 'soft immersion' will be in the brochure, at least as far as small planing craft are concerned.

This is because, when a bow with concave sections becomes immersed, powerful forces start to act upwards against it. Buoyancy increases abruptly at the chine, which hits the water like a board. However a convex section gives rise to braking suction forces and immersion is softer. For example, when the two bow shapes shown opposite are suddenly brought to rest by downward immersion in a wave, bow No 2, with convex sections, lands much more softly than bow No 1. Nevertheless you see quite a few boats with concave bow sections, and not just on older designs. Indeed in the case of large, relatively heavy boats they just can't be totally avoided. To get these to plane at all, a lot of

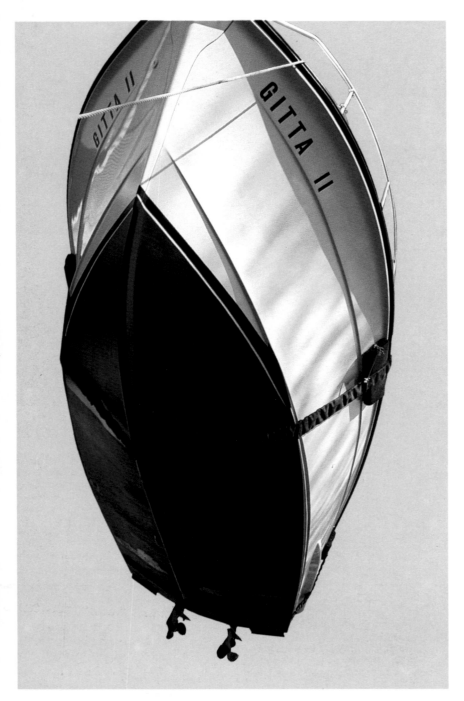

dynamic buoyancy is needed, starting well forward, and a concave forebody provides this.

However, what you can't judge from seeing a boat on dry land is whether the hull design is balanced lengthways so that the bow does not lift sharply when the boat hits a wave at high speed. If, after an unavoidable leap in the air, the boat makes contact again with the water almost simultaneously fore and aft, the 'dropping distance' is less. The hull will run more softly and need less horsepower for the same speed. It will be altogether more easily driven.

It is a widely held but mistaken belief that a boat ploughing through the water with its nose in the air is fast and efficient. Indeed the opposite is the case because that attitude results in a disproportionately high level of frictional resistance. An ideally trimmed, correctly powered boat with a well designed hull lifts itself up almost parallel to the surface, with the nose at most 4° up. This means it is riding almost exclusively on its stern and propeller(s) – fast and relatively

Fast but hard – a typical hull shape from the era before the deep 'V'. Only a moderate deadrise in the forward third of the hull, with the underside towards the stern almost flat. Such boats need less horsepower than those with a more pronounced 'V' and plane relatively quickly. Very dashing when the water is smooth, they feel rock-hard in rough seas. There are still a lot of boats of this early planing type, but few are now being built. The only application for which the shape continues to be suitable is for water-ski boats, where good acceleration and a slight wash are important.

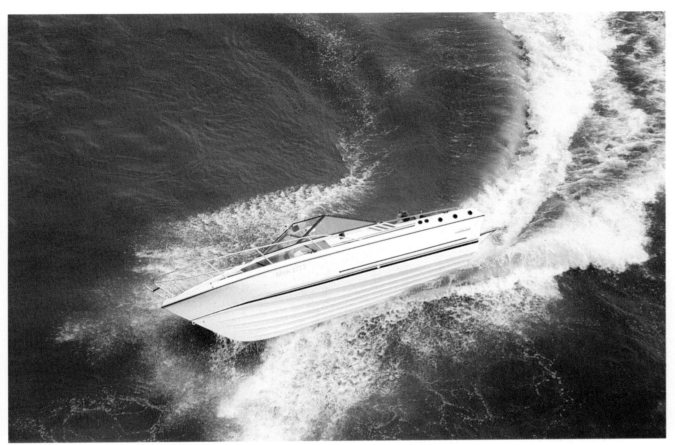

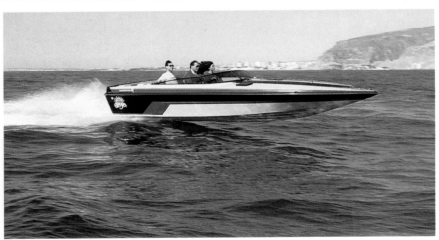

Full-power turn – an 8 metre day cruiser shows her bottom. The modern 'modified V' hull has more deadrise forward but is flatter towards the stern. The moulded external planing stringers increase dynamic lift. These sort of hulls are nowadays so sophisticated that the bow lifts very little when hitting small waves.

The dynamic lift keeps the hull above the water almost parallel to the surface. The retarding wetted surface of the hull is reduced to the minimum, right aft.

gently. Planing craft that spend their time 'trying to climb the stairs' either have an engine that's too heavy or are simply badly designed.

Is the boat going to plane or not?

You can't tell by looking at a boat, particularly one of the larger motor cruisers, whether with the particular engine fitted it is quite such an enthusiastic planer as the brochure and the salesman are trying to make out. If you know the weight of the boat, the reliability of their promises can partly be verified. If a boat with an outdrive or outboard has a weight/power ratio greater than 16.5 kg per hp, it will have trouble planing. For boats with conventional shaft drive the critical boundary is around 22 kg/hp if the hull's aft deadrise is small. A V-bottom, on the other hand, with a deadrise of around 24° along its length, could have difficulty planing at as little as 18 kg/hp. Such heavy, and for their weight, inadequately powered boats, even if they can be persuaded to plane at full power, are unlikely to be able to make a planing passage if speed is reduced to 80% of full revs. They are then stuck on the high-resistance hump and the engine will have a fearful thirst.

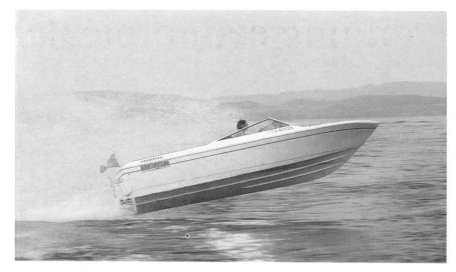

Nose-up leaps in the air are spectacular, but are not good for the crew or for fuel economy.

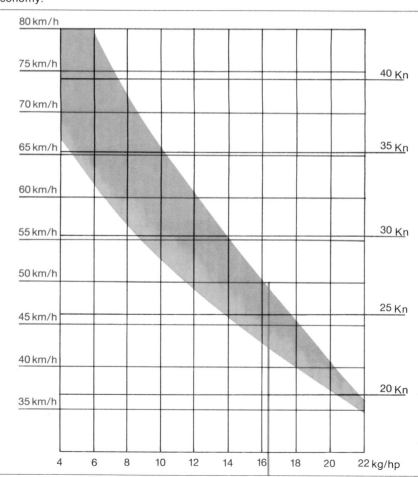

The speed limit for planing craft. The graph shows the approximate speeds to be expected (depending on hull design) with given power : weight ratios in kg/hp. To calculate the power : weight ratio the total weight, ie boat plus engine, full tanks, useful load and passengers, has to be used. The red line through the curve shows the planing limit for outboards and outdrives.

Running economically

Economical running has been mentioned several times, but how are you supposed to known when you are squirting fuel uselessly out of the exhaust pipe?

The most important instrument for establishing this is the rev counter, from which you can tell whether the engine attains its nominal revs, the maximum number given by the manufacturer, at full power. Small divergences from this standard, of the order of 200 to 300 per min, are acceptable; more than that, and you've got the wrong propeller. Reduced to the simplest terms:

Revs too high = prop/pitch too small
Revs too low = prop/pitch too large

For every inch of change in propeller pitch, the revs change by about 200 per min. If you change your propeller, a pitch reduction gives an increase in revs, while a pitch increase gives a reduction in revs. We shall discuss propeller pitch in greater detail later.

Whether an engine is under-revving (not reaching its design revs) or over-revving, it is at any rate running uneconomically and shortening its life expectancy – possibly considerably.

If the nominal revs are about right, the rev counter is an excellent means

of establishing when one is running economically and whether what's in the tank will take you to the next refuelling point. The relationship between engine revs and consumption is pretty well fixed. Using the curve shown here, anyone can estimate what his boat's consumption will be. All you need do is insert the nominal revs of your boat at 100% throttle and the full-power consumption also at 100%. This relationship between engine revs and consumption, which remains the same for most types of engine, derives from the driving characteristics of the propeller.

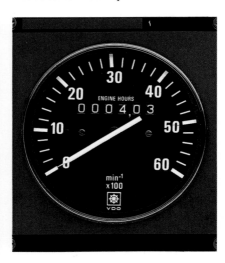

The top priority for power boat instrumentation is the rev counter. This is important for checking the designed (maximum) revs, selecting the right prop, determining the appropriate engine power and the economical speed.

The curve that shows you how to save fuel and money and yet travel fast.

Engine revs %	100	90	70	60	50
Consumption %	100	80	48	34	28

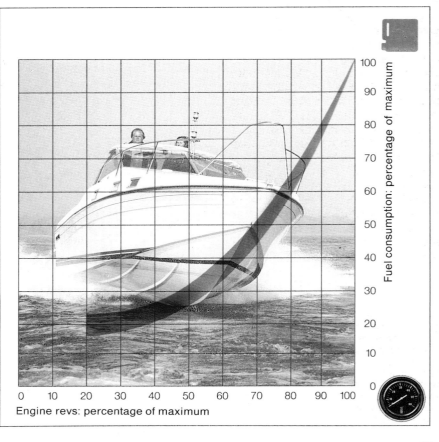

Engine revs: percentage of maximum

Fuel consumption: percentage of maximum

A propeller will absorb power from the engine in proportion to the third exponent of the revs. Boat speed, on the other hand, reduces only proportionally to the revs, at least in the higher rev region. Therefore, pushing the throttle lever(s) hard forward will, particularly with a high-powered planing craft, be a heavy drain on your purse. The increase in speed you get from increasing engine revs becomes less and less the higher the revs.

About 80% of the nominal revs (where fuel consumption reduces to about 60% of maximum) is generally considered a practical maximum cruising speed. 70% of nominal revs (48% of fuel consumption) constitutes a good and economical cruising speed for longer passages, unless a semi-displacement craft is then stuck on the high resistance hump between $R = 5$ and $R = 6.5$. That would mean that it is unquestionably under-engined and running uneconomically, with the consumption no longer sticking to the normal curve but increasing sharply. Obviously even a planing craft has to be pushed over this hump as quickly as possible. That often makes it necessary to go to full power initially and ease off the revs again once you are up on the plane. You can feel when this maximum resistance has been overcome, because the boat lowers its nose again and speeds up noticeably in spite of the revs remaining constant.

For displacement craft economical cruising speed is often at 50% of the nominal revs, with a 72% fuel saving. This increases your effective weather range by at least 100%. Expressed another way, one tankful will take you twice as far.

Planing craft revs can rarely be reduced below 60% of maximum because otherwise the craft would drop into the zone of the high resistance hump. If on the other hand more than 60% are needed to lift the stern out of the water, that is a clear sign that the boat is under-powered. In this connection, another observation is also interesting: for comparable cruising speeds, the revs of a fast-running petrol engine can of course be reduced substantially further than those of a slower-running diesel. Hence it follows that, analogously to our curve, the diesel, much-lauded as being so economical, can swallow just about as much as the petrol engine. This becomes even clearer if you compare the consumption per distance covered (kilometres or nautical miles). Although a petrol engine has a substantially higher litre per hour (ℓ/h) consumption than a diesel, it can nevertheless run equally 'economically'. Assume a boat with a petrol engine has a consumption of 20 ℓ/h at a maximum speed of 50 km/h. Its consumption then is:

$$20\ell/h \div 50 \, km/h = 0.4 \, \ell/km.$$

A diesel-powered boat may have a consumption of 4 ℓ/h at a maximum speed of 10 km/h. Its consumption therefore is:

$$4 \, \ell/h \div 10 \, km/h = 0.4 \, \ell/km.$$

Admittedly, to accept this kind of economy, you have to have a liking for leisurely meandering afloat.

How far is the fuel going to go?

Running economically not only concerns the wallet but also affects actually 'getting there'. We have already briefly mentioned range. It is often confused with radius of action – and that is fatal! For the radius of action is only half the range, ie a position from which with the available fuel in the tank you can safely return to your point of departure.

The first move when going to sea – or travelling on a river for that matter – is passage planning and therefore the question: how many kilometres or nautical miles can I cover with a full tank? Here we need first of all to consider the consumption of the various types of engine at full power (ie at nominal revs).

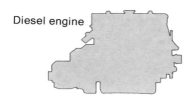

Diesel engine

Direct injection	0.20 ℓ/Hph (0.27 ℓ/kW
Indirect injection	0.25 ℓ/Hph (0.34 ℓ/kW

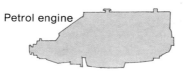

Petrol engine

Four stroke	0.30 ℓ/Hph (0.41 ℓ/kW

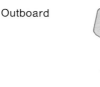

Outboard

Two-stroke	0.40 ℓ/Hph (0.54 ℓ/kW

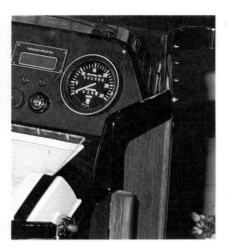

A boat speedometer or log indicating knots (nautical miles per hour) or kilometres per hour, with counters for total, daily, or trip distance covered. In combination with the rev counter, the log is a valuable aid to route planning and fuel consumption measurement.

Exceptions, by up to as much as 15%, occasionally occur in the case of outboards, but they are anyway not significant in this connection. The calculation is relatively simple: the full-power hp (kW) × 0.30 (0.41) or × 0.25 (0.34), depending on whether the engine is a petrol or a diesel one, gives the hourly consumption. It now depends on the capacity of your tank how many hours it allows you to cruise around. And it depends on the rev-related speed – indicated by the speedometer – how far you can get in that time.

Assuming our boat has a tank of 400 litre capacity, a 200 hp indirect-injection diesel and can do 52 km/h: A calculation shows:

200 hp × 0.25 ℓ/h = 50 ℓ/h
400 ℓ : 50 ℓ/h = 8 h
8 h × 52 km = 416 km.

With a full tank we can in 8 hours cover a distance of 416 km at full power. But since you wouldn't inflict that either on yourself or on the engine, but rather would travel at perhaps 75% of the full power revs, you always automatically have a certain distance-left-to-go in the tank. All the same, when planning any passage you should select staging points such that even running at full speed you would still arrive with a 10% reserve in the tank – just in case of emergencies. And you need to add at least another 10% reserve, because if the sea is rough, about 10% of the tank contents can't be used.

Let's do another sample calculation:

A boat capable of 60 km/h fitted with a 120 hp petrol engine at full power consumes 36 ℓ/h. We reduce the revs to 70%. The speed also comes down to about 70% (42 km/h) but the consumption drops to about 48% (17.3 ℓ/h). Since our boat at full power does 60 km/h, it uses 0.6 ℓ per kilometre. At 42 km/h, only 0.4 ℓ/km. The same amount of fuel is now enough for about a 46% longer passage. That can be a vital factor at sea. If you suddenly discover that you're getting short of fuel and decide to hurry to reach the next bunkering point, you probably won't make it. Only by going fairly slowly will you reach the destination.

A motor yacht at sea can, at any time, meet unexpected heavy weather. Maybe on that account her skipper will decide to make for an alternative port much farther off than the original destination for which the fuel reserve was calculated. Throttling back to

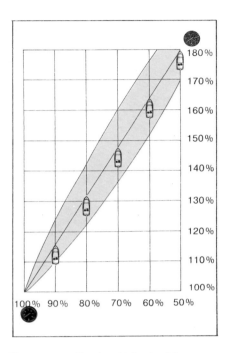

How many miles are in the tank?
100% ℓ/min = fuel consumption at your maximum revs
100% km(nm) = your range on one tankful at maximum revs

This graph gives you some idea of how far you can get at what revs on one tankful, so long as you know your full power consumption by measurement or calculation. If you reduce the revs from the design figure to 50% the range (distance you can cover) increases by up to 80% or theoretically even by 100%. However, owing to the retarding and power consuming influence of wind, current and waves these increases are not obtained in practice. If planing craft slow down to displacement speed, consumption may increase disproportionately. The calculation doesn't necessarily apply to outboards either, whose consumption is unpredictable in the lower rev range.

half power increases the range by about 80%: eg from 30 km to 540. In most cases, that will be enough to ensure arrival. But watch it! There's something else that has to be taken into account in rough weather: high winds and heavy seas are exceedingly power-consuming in themselves. Fuel consumption in the upper power region, ie at 80 to 90% of nominal revs, can just about double. The contents of your tank are suddenly only enough for half the distance. Scarcely anyone is aware of this so should you by any chance get caught out you could run into serious trouble by being short of fuel.

But it isn't just wind and weather which can upset your calculations. Boat hulls sitting still in the water for long periods tend to accumulate patches of weed and barnacles. These can increase frictional resistance by up to 20% and increase consumption correspondingly. The first sign that you're dragging something along on your underside is that the engine no longer reaches its previous revs.

What consumption-checks reveal

The figures in these three tables are based on averages from dozens of tests of all currently popular sizes of motor boats fitted with a variety of engines. The readings for the pure displacement craft are very typical. The minimum consumption and maximum range are right at the lowest working revs. As engine speed increases, these values increase/decrease progressively. Semi-displacement craft mostly have a noticeable break in fuel consumption (here at 2100 rpm) at the economical

speed where the hull begins to lift out of the water – though the consumption is still greater and the range less than the lowest working revs.

The planing craft has the most noticeable break where it has started to plane (here at 3000 rpm). The boat achieves its longest range and minimum consumption at its lowest planing speed. Running more slowly, in the displacement mode, consumption goes up and range down.

Characteristic measured values   ☐ **Economical speed**

Engine rpm	Speed (knots)	Consumption (litres per nm)	Max range on a full tank (nm)
No 1 Displacement craft, waterline length 10.75/R = 5.1			
1500	4.7	1.19	1012
2000	6.0	1.35	754
2500	7.0	1.69	605
3000	8.0	2.32	440
3500	8.5	3.44	295
4000	9.1	4.65	219
No 2 Semi-displacement craft, waterline length 10.75/R = 12.9			
1000	6.9	3.19	289
1400	8.5	3.43	270
1800	8.9	4.43	209
2100	14.6	3.50	264
2400	18.0	4.06	228
2900	22.9	6.02	153
No 3 Planing craft, waterline length 8.70/R = 24.9			
1000	5.0	1.63	156
1500	7.2	1.81	140
2500	16.0	1.80	142
3000	23.9	1.54	165
3500	28.3	1.74	146
4000	32.4	2.00	127
4200	34.1	2.09	122

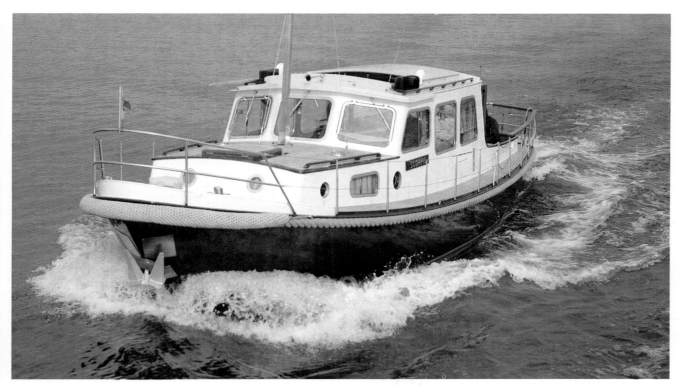

What running records reveal about consumption and power

Back to economical running and the question of the right engine to fit. Let's consider the meaning in practice of what has been said so far, using real boats as examples. Precise consumption and speed measurements form the basis of this analysis; you can deduce a lot from these figures.

Displacement craft Valkvlet
Length overall .... 10.30 metres
Waterline length .... 9.00 metres
Beam .... 3.30 metres
Weight (displacement) .... 10 tonnes
Hull speed .... 13.5 km/h
Engine: 106 hp (78 kW) Ford diesel

Results of the measurement runs with the Valkvet (displacement craft)

Revs		Speed	Consumption			Range on 1 full tank	Running time of 1 full tank
1/min	%*	km/h	l/km	l/h	%*	(400 l) km**	h:min
2500	100	15.3	1.93	29.5	100	176	11:30
2000	80	13.5	1.30	17.5	59	262	19:07
1500	60	12.0	0.67	8.4	29	507	42:15
1000	40	8.3	0.35	2.9	10	971	116.59

*Rounded up/down to whole% **Less 15% reserve   ▢ Economical speed

This steel-hulled motor yacht is a typical displacement craft with a traditional round bilge hull. It attains its theoretical hull speed of 13.5 km/h at 80% of the nominal revs. The boat is comparatively strongly powered for a displacement craft, so has sufficient spare power to deal with even a fast-flowing current. The economical speed is reached using only 40% of the nominal revs. In the rev region below 60%, the ℓ/km consumption is unusually low. These data indicate careful matching of engine and propeller to the boat type. Even a few horsepower less could easily be justified.

Heavy planing craft Conti 305
Length overall .... 9.25 metres
Waterline length .... 7.65 metres
Beam .... 3.00 metres
Weight (displacement) ... 4.9 tonnes
Hull speed .... 12.4 km/h
Engine: 2 × 165 hp (121 kW) Volvo
            Penta Aquamatic (diesel)

This comparatively heavy seagoing motor cruiser has a rather feeble engine. You can see how, around 2000 revs, it is labouring to overcome the high resistance (R = 5.4). The ℓ/km consumption leaps up; the range drops like a stone. The economical cruising speed is reached at 3100 rpm, shortly after the boat has started to plane. Not a lot of spare power is left in the upper rev region. It would be a good idea to fit the next higher-power engine on offer, or possible lighter petrol engines of similar power. (The consumption given in the table for one engine must of course be doubled for the two.)

Results of the fuel measurement runs with the Conti 305 (heavy planing craft)

Revs		Speed	Consumption			Range on 1 full tank	Running time of 1 full tank
1/min	%*	km/h	l/km	l/h	%*	(600 l) km**	h:min
3600	100	49.4	0.78	38.5	100	327	6:37
3400	94	46.3	0.72	33.3	87	354	7:39
3100	86	38.4	0.70	26.9	70	364	9:29
2800	78	29.7	0.71	21.0	55	359	12.05
2000	56	14.8	0.88	13.0	34	290	19:36
1600	44	12.3	0.73	9.0	23	349	28:22

*Rounded up/down to whole %   **Less 15% reserve   [ ] Economical speed

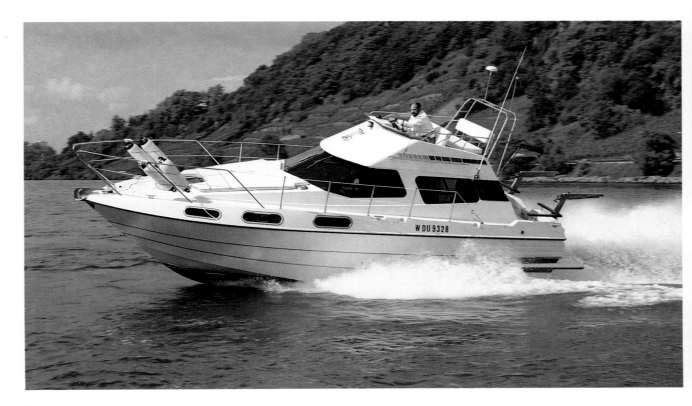

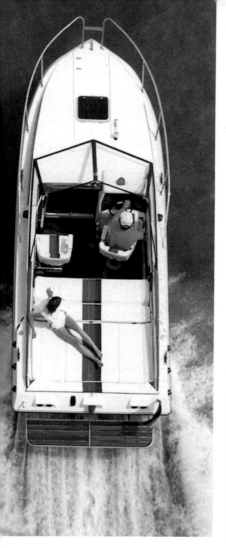

Planing craft Seacruiser 790
Length overall .... 7.90 metres
Waterline length .... 6.85 metres
Beam .... 2.50 metres
Weight (displacement) ... 1870 kilo-
                            grammes
Engine: 270 hp (199 kW) Volvo Penta
                  Aquamatic (petrol)

Unquestionably a planing craft, the Seacruiser slots somewhere between day-cruisers and cabin boats. That it is slightly over-engined you can see from the fact that it's already planing fully at less than 50% nominal revs. This is shown by the way the speed leaps up between 2000 and 2500 revs, while simultaneously the ℓ/km consumption drops by nearly a half. Economical cruising speed (lowest ℓ/km consumption and thus maximum range) is reached at a mere 64% of the nominal revs. Consumption then drops to 42% of maximum. To dash about faster than that would be extravagant. Such an excess of power is advantageous in that it means a relatively low fuel consumption at high speed. It is at any rate more economical – leaving aside the first

cost of the engine – than if you just manage to reach planing speed with an insufficiently powerful engine running near the top of its rev-range. Also you always have a sufficient reserve of power if wind and waves were to force you to reduce speed. This boat, so the measurement data prove, is right in all practical respects: design, weight, engine power and propeller.

Let us finally take another look at the reduction curve on which the readings from these three boats have been plotted. Three totally different engine installations and boat types, but they all stay precisely on the line – only the Ford diesel shows a drop near the bottom end, although that might equally well be due to some imprecision in the measurements.

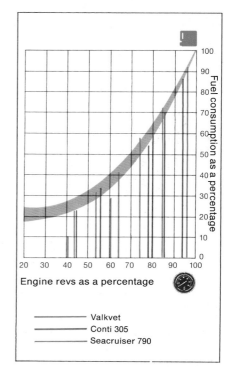

Results of the fuel measurement runs with the Seacruiser 790 (planing craft)

Revs		Speed	Consumption			Range on 1 full tank	Running time of 1 full tank
1/min	%*	km/h	l/km	l/h	%*	(200 l) km**	h:min
4700	100	76.5	1.15	87.9	100	148	1:56
4500	96	73.5	1.11	81.6	93	153	2:05
4000	85	64.5	1.00	64.5	73	170	2:38
3500	74	55.7	0.91	50.7	58	187	3:21
3000	64	44.9	0.82	36.8	42	207	4:37
2500	53	34.1	0.84	28.6	32	202	5:55
2000	43	13.2	1.56	20.6	23	109	8:15

*Rounded up/down to whole % **Less 15% reserve ☐ Economical speed

The heart of the motor boat – the power unit

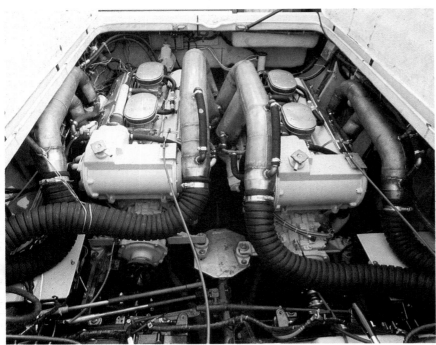

Inboard engines must have a good air supply, and accessibility for checking and maintenance. Many engine compartments are badly off in both respects, particularly if two engines have to share a compartment originally intended for one. Every engine compartment should, as far as possible, be lined with sound absorbing, non-flammable material.

Almost all boat engines – except for the specially-developed outboard motors – are based on tried and proven car or industrial engines. However to marinise these basic blocks calls for extensive modification. Most of the effort is required for the water cooling circuit and the exhaust system with their mass of niggly technical details. Added to this is the awkward to fit reduction and reverse gearing, and the heavy duty spark-proof starter and generator, so that you find that a marine engine finally shows only a distant kinship with its automotive counterpart. When everything about the design is right, the engine still has to be prop-

erly installed in the boat, with its mounting points firmly anchored on rubber/metal bearers. Many a boat engine is short of breath in its narrow, maintenance-impeding 'engine room', and for that reason alone it may never achieve the promised output; losses may be up to 15% of theoretical power. As on the road, there are petrol and diesel engines. Let us briefly recall the significant differences: petrol engines suck in a petrol-air mixture through the carburettor which is ignited by an electric spark plug. Diesels suck in only air, which is heated so much by strong compression that the injected diesel oil ignites spontaneously. So the diesel has no carburet-

tor and no electric ignition system; instead it has a fuel pump and fuel injectors. The petrol engine is switched off with the ignition key, the diesel with a stop-button which interrupts the fuel supply.

Both systems have their advantages and disadvantages. A diesel is more expensive to buy, and the higher first cost can barely be made good by its 30% lower consumption in the few running hours which a boat engine accumulates in a season. But a diesel also needs less maintenance because it has fewer parts susceptible to failure. It thus has a longer life – workshop experts talk of 50%. But the decisive argument put forward by protagonists is that a diesel engine in a boat is substantially safer than a petrol engine. A petrol engine produces dangerous vapours which, when mixed with air and ignited by a spark, can cause an explosion even at $-25°C$ (ie in practice at any time); however, with a diesel, that risk arises only above $+55°C$. Furthermore, a diesel has no sparking components. In return for the added safety and reliability, one is happy to accept the greater weight, larger overall dimensions, and increased noise and vibration.

The principal argument for the better-value-for-money, more highly developed and compact petrol engine is its favourable power-to-weight ratio. This is calculated by dividing the weight of the engine by its output in hp or kW. Basically one can say that the higher the engine revs, the lower or more favourable is its power to weight ratio. A low power-to weight ratio for a long time blocked the slow-running diesel's entry into the engine compartments of planing craft. However technical progress produced fast-running diesels with

The petrol engine – the trimmings which marinise a car engine. Only what is clearly visible is identified here; many refinements are concealed.

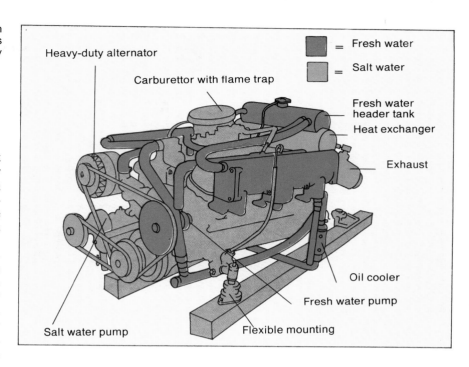

Heavy-duty alternator

Carburettor with flame trap

= Fresh water

= Salt water

Fresh water header tank

Heat exchanger

Exhaust

Oil cooler

Fresh water pump

Flexible mounting

Salt water pump

more favourable power-to-weight ratios, and the turbocharger rapidly captured the field for diesel engines in boats. It raised the ratio so substantially from its low level that there are few craft today in which petrol engines are fitted on weight grounds.

Do you remember how the turbocharger, whose exclusion from the boat propulsion field would now be quite unthinkable, actually works? The exhaust drives a turbine and this in turn a blower which draws in air and raises the pressure at which it enters the cylinders. This makes more oxygen available for combustion, allowing more fuel to be injected. Result: power increases, the fuel is burnt more completely, and specific consumption is reduced. If a charge cooler is added, power increases even further: it cools the air, (heated by being compressed) down again before discharging it to the cylinders. However there are also disadvantages to be recorded: in the low and medium rev range the turbine efficiency is low and the control of fuel injection has its problems.

Direct-injection diesels have fuel injected directly into a cavity in the cylinder. These are the most economical engines, and the noisiest.

Indirect-injection engines, in which the fuel is ignited in a precombustion or swirl chamber, swallow about 25% more and need a heater plug for cold starting. Amongst the petrol engines

there are two-strokes and four-strokes, the principal difference being that the two-stroke operates with a petrol-oil mixture which provides the necessary lubrication. The four-stroke burns pure petrol; an oil pump feeds oil from a separate sump to all parts requiring lubrication. The two-stroke gets its oil, in the correct proportion, fed into the fuel tank and that's all. The four-stroke on the other hand needs conscientious oil monitoring and the oil changed at intervals which are laid down in the operating manual; usually a hundred running hours. Running an engine with oil that is too old can incur bearing damage if the oil film breaks down.

Almost all inboard engines are four-strokes, almost all outboards are two-strokes. The two-strokes may be the thirstiest, but they have their

advantages: compactness and low weight because valves, pushrods, oil pumps and other accessories are eliminated. From the same basic capacity, they'll produce more power than four-strokes.

For displacement craft the diesel is the better power unit. For 8 to 12 metre length cruisers, both diesel and petrol engines are available; bigger boats are predominantly diesel-powered.

Outboard engines

Two-stroke outboard engines for a long time suffered under the stigma of being dirty and not standing up to sea water very well. Acrid bluish clouds of exhaust smoke surrounded early outboards running with a petrol/oil mixture of 10:1 or 25:1. Those smokey machines belong to the past since mixture ratios of 50:1 to 100:1 have become common for outboards. In certain engines, the ratio may be as little as 150:1. 'Self-mixing' oil is added in the correct proportion to the petrol in the tank. With technically more sophisticated engines, the oil is fed from a separate tank by a pump or injected under microprocessor control. This is the cleanest, and for combustion quality an ideal, solution.

Outboards are now much better encapsulated against moisture and are generally just as reliable and efficient as inboard engines.

The range of outboards extends from 2 hp (1.5 kW) up to more than 200 hp (150 kW). The lower powered ones are started by hand using a starter cord; the larger ones are started electrically using an ignition key. For power-to-weight, the outboard is unbeatable; no inboard engine can get anywhere near it. It is the ideal power unit for all open sports boats.

How do you find the engine that matches your boat? There is a curve, somewhat modified but based on the many years of experience of the American Boating Industry Association. It was worked out to safeguard drivers of outboard-engined boats against fitting too much horsepower and thus endangering themselves and others. It shows the maximum power for normal planing craft and drivers

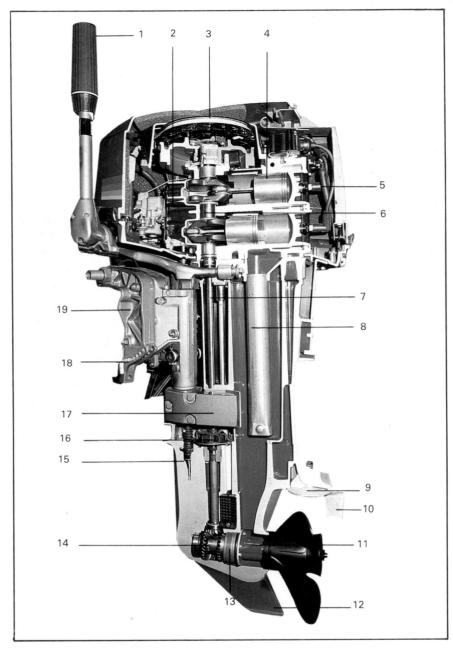

An outboard engine has lots of cunning technology in a compact unit.

1 Tiller with rotary throttle (smaller engines up to about 30 hp only). 2 Carburettor. 3 Flywheel. 4 Cylinder (a 2-cylinder engine). 5 Spark plugs. 6 Crankshaft. 7 Drive shaft. 8 Exhaust duct. 9 Cavitation plate with cooling water outlet. 10 Trim tab for balancing paddle wheel effect. 11 Exhaust aperture in propeller hub. 12 Skeg (protects the prop). 13 Prop shaft. 14 Bevel gear and clutch. 15 Gear shift linkage (the lower part which engages the gear is not shown in this sectional view). 16 Cooling water pump. 17 Lower shaft bearing. 18 Tilt-adjusting holes with socket pins. 19 Tilting bracket (locking arrangement beneath).

experienced with throttle and wheel. Beginners should make do with half or three quarters of the indicated horsepower; the boat will nevertheless plane perfectly. The maximum power is recommended and appropriate if the boat is to be used a lot for water-skiing.

The great advantage of outboard engines is their portability. Outboards up to a certain size can easily be removed from the boat for security,

taken home in the car boot or driven to your local engineer's workshop for servicing. It is also relatively easy to change an outboard engine, perhaps for a more powerful model, although large outboards, while self-contained, are also very heavy. A 100 hp (73 kW) engine can easily weigh 150 kg (330 lb) and could only be lifted on and off the boat safely with a small crane. For trailable boats with large outboards, it's usually easier to haul the boat out

with the engine still attached and trail the whole outfit to the workshop for servicing.

Although larger outboards can have amazingly high horsepower, they are really only suitable for relatively light boats and high speeds. The engines are high revving and have small diameter propellers, a combination which is geared for speed and not power. When fitted to slower, heavier boats, powerful outboards have a poor efficiency, so you cannot directly compare the 150 hp of a racing outboard and the 150 hp (110 kW) of a six cylinder diesel engine driving a displacement motor yacht.

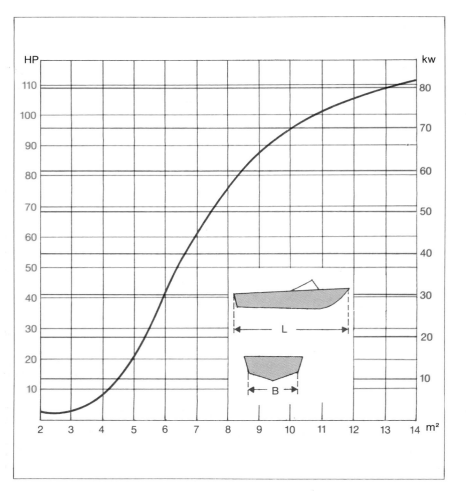

This helps you find the right outboard for your boat. The boat size is calculated from the overall length and the width of the transom at the waterline. For example: 4.70 m long × 1.80 m wide = 8.46 m². Maximum engine power for this would be 85 hp (63 kW); recommended power would be 60–70 hp.

Engine transmissions

Most marine engine transmission systems use mechanical gearing of some kind. Hydraulic transmissions are only used for specialized applications, being comparatively expensive and inefficient in terms of power loss. The main purpose of the transmission system is to transfer the power output from the engine to the propeller, which finally drives the boat. However, the transmission has to incorporate three other functions as well:

- A reversing facility, so that the propeller can be either driven ahead, declutched into 'neutral', or reversed for going astern.
- A reduction gearing, so that the relatively high revs of the engine are geared down to lower revs for driving the propeller.
- A thrust bearing, which absorbs the lengthwise driving thrust, either ahead or astern, which the propeller generates in the prop shaft.

The fixed shaft drive

This is often called the 'conventional' shaft drive because it used to be the only drive available for yachts. The prop shaft slopes down inside a stern tube through the boat's bottom, below which it may be supported by a shaft bracket. If the engine crankshaft, gearing and shaft all lie in the same plane this is called an L- (= line) drive. If there is a more or lesss acute angle between crank and prop shaft and they act in opposite directions, the installation is known as V-drive. The

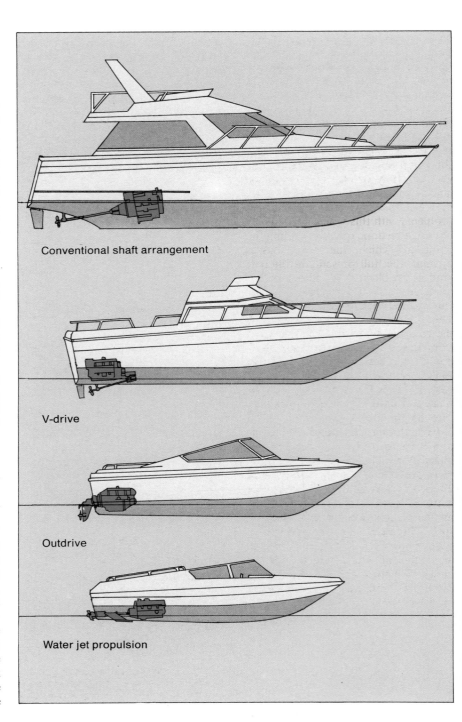

Conventional shaft arrangement

V-drive

Outdrive

Water jet propulsion

direction change is effected via universal joints or bevel wheels and two gearwheels. In this way, the engine can be installed close to and above, or even further aft than, the propeller. There are times when this makes good sense, allowing better use of the space in the boat or to improve its trim.

In conventional installations, prop shaft and engine have to be aligned very carefully or else you'll soon be landed with bearing damage. It can't be denied that yards occasionally have problems with this work, particularly if it must be done quickly. Sealing the point at which the shaft passes through the hull presents a different kind of problem. A gland prevents – or at least should prevent – water entering the boat along the prop shaft. The gland packing, pressing against the rotating shaft, must be adjusted from time to time so that the shaft doesn't run completely dry, but also so that as little water as possible leaks past. It needs frequent checking and there is usually a grease gun to lubricate the gland.

Even today, 'conventional' shaft drives are the only practicable installations for yachts more than about 11 metres long and engines of more than 290 hp (215 kW). But they are also the most effective for smaller displacement craft that don't exceed their hull speed, because they combine with a pusher-propeller of largish diameter and efficient characteristics. Boats under 11 metres with less than about 290 horsepower are often powered by outdrives.

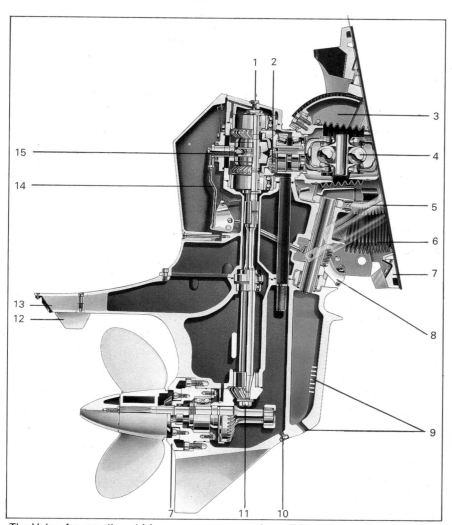

The Volvo Aquamatic outdrive.
1 Oil dipstick for the outdrive unit
2 1st bevel gear
3 Steering casing encloses the universal joint shaft
4 Universal joint in drive shaft, permits tilting/steering with outdrive
5 Tilting cylinder for altering the angle of the Aquamatic
6 Rubber bellows, exhaust duct from the engine into the shaft
7 Zinc anodes as corrosion protection
8 Tilting release for obstructions; also astern lock preventing drive unit from tilting upwards if astern power is applied too quickly
9 Cooling water inlet
10 Oil drain for the outdrive unit
11 2nd bevel gear to the prop shaft
12 Trim tab balances paddlewheel effect
13 Cavitation plate with exhaust and cooling water outlets
14 Gear change linkage, allows prop direction of rotation to be changed by over-centre movement
15 Cone clutch for going ahead and astern

Just like the outboard, the outdrive has a spring-loaded catch that opens only if the submerged portion collides with an obstacle. This protects the outdrive and prop from damage, at least at slow speed.

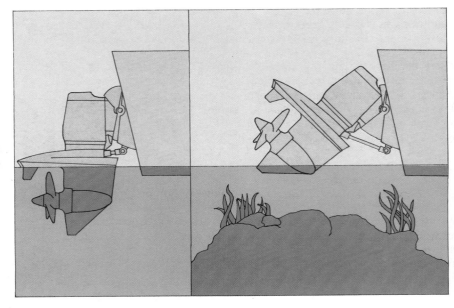

The outdrive

This type of transmission is sometimes called 'Aquamatic' after the name of the prototype from the Swedish engine builder Volvo Penta. The outboard element fastened to the transom is connected to the drive shaft by a universal joint. The drive is turned through a right angle at the head of the (outboard) shaft and engages the tail shaft, at right angles again, via bevel gears.

Steering is direct, using the swivel and tiltable outboard element. This makes for much more positive manoeuvring than with a rudder behind a fixed shaft drive. Installing such a unit in a boat is relatively straightforward because engine and transmission constitute one compact assembly. All that's needed is a carefully cut opening in the transom, through which the Aquamatic is mounted. This system just about halves installation time, and thus also the cost. There is no need for the complicated cooling water piperuns and exhaust cooling of the fixed shaft drive. The outdrive pumps up the cooling water it needs through its submerged portion and discharges it again with the exhaust gases.

The advantages of being able to tilt up the Aquamatic are considerable: you can ground the boat to step ashore comfortably; check at once if

something has fouled the propeller; remove plastic bags, ropes or weed; change the propeller without having to lift the boat out of the water. When lifting the boat by crane, there's no need to fear damage from the lifting gear to shaft or propeller. It's also much easier to stow your boat on the trailer and transport it. Propellers are less vulnerable to damage because the outdrive – just like an outboard – tilts up if it encounters an underwater obstacle, at least when going slowly. As with large outboards, a hydraulic system called 'power-trim' permits continuous adjustment of the outdrive leg's angle of attack.

Most inboard engined sports boats and day cruisers up to about 11 metres in length are fitted with outdrives. In contrast to the fixed shaft transmission, the outdrive does not transmit its thrust to the main part of the hull directly but via the propeller leg and the stern. To prevent problems in the transmission of large torsional and

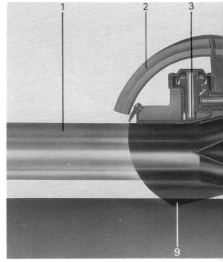

A Castoldi water jet drive.

1 Expelled jet of water
2 Deflector (reversing scoop) for controlling going ahead/astern
3 Shaft for rotating the two rudder blades at the nozzle outlet
4 Inspection flap for the impeller chamber

compression forces, without involving heavyweight technology in the outdrive and its mountings, torque is kept to a minimum by using small propellers and high revs. Such propellers would not be suitable for heavier and slower boats and so the outdrive system is naturally limited to faster, lighter ones.

Jet propulsion

Water-jet propulsion is sometimes regarded as a rather exotic or futuristic means of driving motor boats, although it is being used increasingly for luxury yachts. The water or hydro-jet drive dispenses with reversing gear, prop and rudder and instead the engine drives an impeller in a pump casing. Water drawn in through a duct in the boat's bottom is accelerated and ejected at high pressure through the driving jet nozzle. You steer by deflecting the jet with a flap or by swivelling the jet at the stern. The jet-drive system calls for its own driving technique, which we shall consider later. Its efficiency is about 10% less than that of propeller drive, sometimes up to 50% less at slow speeds. Jet drives are often fitted to rescue craft because there are no parts of the drive projecting below the bottom, which could be easily damaged or cause injury.

Neither too hot nor too cold – the cooling system

Like almost all outboards, most inboard engines are water-cooled. Some open work boats use air-cooled engines, but it is difficult to install ducts large enough to provide an adequate amount of cooling air on boats. There are two types of water-cooling systems: single-circuit cooling – also called direct or raw-water cooling; and dual-circuit or heat-exchange cooling. Single-circuit cooling systems pump in water via a seacock, circulate it continuously through the engine's water jacket, and discharge it overboard again, usually through the exhaust system. Direct cooling takes up a minimum of space, and installation and maintenance are simple, but for seagoing use it has a real disadvantage. At temperatures above about 65°C, the seawater deposits calcium and sodium salts, which can build up to restrict and eventually block the cooling passages in the engine. To avoid that happening, the engine has to be run too cold, at well below its design temperature. The temperature at which most engines really 'feel well' is between 80° and 90°C. Running much cooler than this results in reduced efficiency, higher fuel consumption, and also more rapid wear because the lower temperature additionally makes engine lubrication less effective. Perhaps more important is the risk that, should cooling break down, because of a pump defect or a blocked water inlet, the almost instantaneous rise in temperature can very quickly damage the engine seriously.

With dual-circuit cooling, the engine is cooled by a closed fresh water circuit, driven by its own pump.

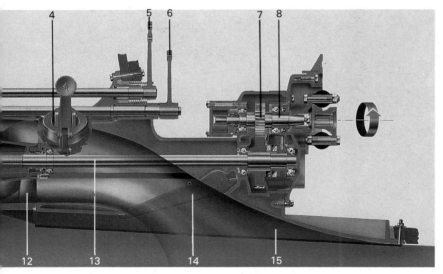

5	Connection for the control cable to the deflector shaft
6	Connection for the control cable to the rudder shaft
7	Clutch
8	Drive shaft (from engine)
9	Rudder blades for deflecting jet sideways
0	Conical convergent jet nozzle
11	Impeller casing
12	Three-bladed impeller (axial flow wheel)
13	Impeller shaft
14	Protective grating with removable rods for cleaning
15	Intake duct (part of outboard element)

The fresh water is cooled in a heat exchanger mounted on the engine, a compact system of tubes through which sea or river water is pumped from outside the boat. A thermostat opens as soon as the required operating temperature has been reached. In this way the engine can always be operated efficiently within its designed temperature range. Should a breakdown occur, because of a pump inpeller failing or the seacock becoming blocked by a plastic bag, the engine temperature rises only gradu-

ally, and the fault should be detected in good time by the engine instruments. The space requirement is of course greater, and the system with its heat exchanger, fresh water tank and second pump is more sophisticated and accordingly more expensive. Surface cooling systems also incorporate a closed fresh water circuit.

Using the hull surface for cooling is of course only practicable with steel hulls. The cooling passages are in direct contact with the steel outer skin, which transfers the heat to the sur-

rounding water. Keel-tube cooling, which uses pipes mounted on or near the keel, works on the same principle. You sometimes find this in steel hulled displacement yachts. However, if the water temperature is high and the boat's speed low – eg with both wind and sea against you – the rate of heat removal may be inadequate.

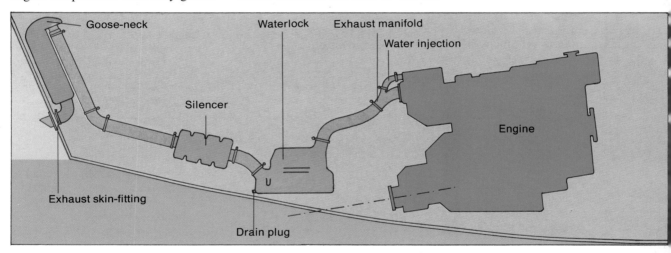

A wet exhaust system cooled by the engine cooling water. When the engine is stopped, the water in the system collects in the waterlock. If the engine is below the waterline, the cooling system must be vented with a siphon-break to prevent water running back to the engine.

With single circuit (raw-water) cooling, sea water (blue) is pumped directly through the engine cooling jacket (left). With dual-circuit cooling, the sea water flows through a heat exchanger and cools the fresh water (green) in the inner, closed, circuit. Outdrives draw in cooling water through the shaft and discharge it through the shaft with the exhaust.

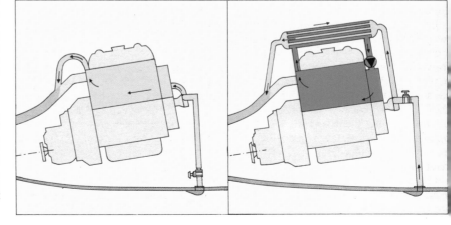

Air for the engine to breathe – engine compartment ventilation

An engine can't live without air. A four-stroke needs at least four times its piston displacement to keep the temperature around it reasonable; a rule sinned against more often than not.

An engine that doesn't get enough air drinks too much, suffers from lube-oil dilution, has its plugs soot up and soon will be difficult to start. An intake-air temperature of 20°C is ideal but is seldom attained. At 30°C you already have 5% power loss; at 40°C the loss can be 10%.

The builder will probably have calculated the bare combustion air requirement correctly. The rule of thumb is that engines need 100 litres of air per minute. This is not enough, however, if the engine itself is short of space. This sin of construction is committed more frequently in the case of open boats fitted with outdrives, because builders usually like to keep the engine box small for visual and space reasons.

Lack of air can be the reason why an engine, though matched to its propeller, does not attain its nominal revs. You can establish this by running a trial: if the revs drop at the end of a somewhat prolonged run at full power, without any recognisable cause, this is very probably because the engine has got too hot. If you carry on running with the engine box lid open and the engine then reaches and maintains its full revs again, that is your proof.

Generators and V-belts also suffer if the engine compartment temperature is too high.

One engine or two – does doubling-up pay?

It's not all that long ago that outboard-engined boats were often fitted with two engines, the argument being that this would double their speed and give an additional margin of safety. Two engines would be unlikely to break down at the same time, or go on strike together. This is true enough, but a properly-maintained modern outboard is a very reliable machine which very rarely lets you down. The same arguments can also be applied to outdrives and traditional shaft drives.

If two engines are being considered, the first question is whether the object is to halve the output or to double it. Whether, let's say, 100 hp is to be divided into 2×50 hp or whether another 1×100 hp is to be added. The shared output brings nothing but disadvantages, apart from the safety aspect.

Firstly, a small engine costs more to buy per hp than a large one. Expressed differently: for instance, 250 hp in one unit costs substantially less than 2×120 hp. Secondly the two halves will weigh 20% to 30% more than the whole. Extra weight that needs extra power to push it along. A planing craft with outdrive built for a single engine may well have room for two and a second hole can be cut in the transom – but it may then no longer reach planing speed, or do so only just. Thirdly a larger engine is thermo-mechanically more efficient than any smaller one can be; it thus swallows less fuel per hp. Fourthly a larger centreline propeller attains a much higher efficiency and produces more speed than two smaller off-centre

props for the same nominal engine power. Two shafts also just about double the frictional resistance in the water. All this adds up to a potential speed loss of 10 to 20%. Finally maintenance and inspection of two units doubles the running cost.

Anyone thinking of 'doubling upwards' with the second engine, say from 125 hp to 250, won't double the speed by that means, as is widely believed. That again is due to the interplay of forces involving increased frictional resistance, mutual interference and complex hydrodynamics. At most the second engine gives 30% more speed, and no conscientious engine supplier will promise more than that. But if we make a single engine push out that 250 hp, the boat will run a good 33% faster than with two 125 hp engines. The reasons are

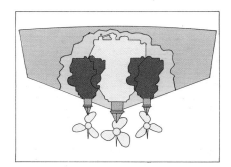

Wide or tall? The large single bulk of, for example, a 275 hp outdrive would stick right up into the cockpit. The twin installation of 140 hp each, on the other hand, fits neatly underneath the sunbathing deck.

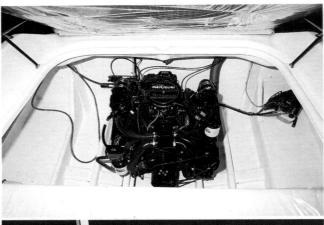
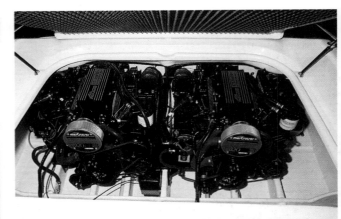
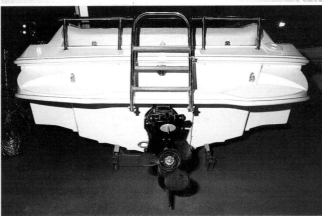
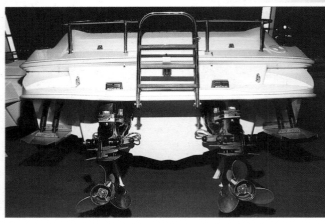

A 7.6 metre day cruiser where the object is to double the engine output (1 × 270 hp/2 × 260 hp). Yet there seems no justifiable relationship between the increased cost and consumption and the 20% increase in maximum speed that could be expected – usable anyway only in dead smooth water. The cramped conditions in the engine compartment make maintenance difficult, and the increased weight aft (here some 600 kg more) can only be compensated for by trim tabs, which often means a narrowing of the economical planing band.

the higher efficiency of the single propeller on the one hand and the reduced resistance of a single shaft.

However, most boatbuilders have good reasons for installing twin engines, the most compelling of which is that they are popular with customers. Twin engines are still perceived as being much safer than a single engine, and they certainly make manoeuvring much simpler. There is a sign of a move back towards single engines for smaller displacement boats, principally on the grounds of cost, and this trend may continue if fuel costs start to rise again.

Engine controls

Anyone who thinks he can transfer to the boat what he is accustomed to doing in the car has a surprise coming: there are no gears to change. Controlling a boat *seems* much simpler, and yet, in practice, it is much more complicated. The boat transmission – no matter what type of engine – has only three control positions: **ahead – neutral – astern**. Lever forwards = travel ahead, lever back = travel astern.

In the case of the still widely fitted two-lever control, the throttle and gear shift are controlled separately. Push the throttle lever forwards and the carburettor opens on the petrol engine, the injection-pump output increases on the diesel. However, before shifting gear, you have to throttle back to idling speed, or else there is a risk of damaging the gearbox and transmission.

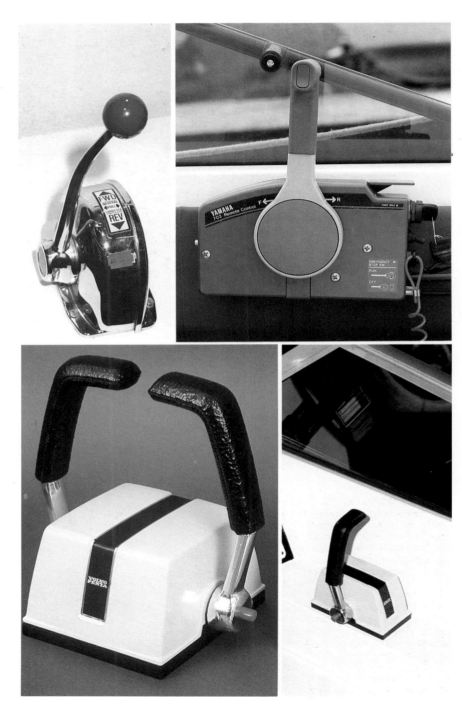

Top left: The original Morse single lever control – probably used more than any other.
Bottom left: single lever control for twin engines and console-mounting. By pressing in the red button, the lever operates the throttle only – useful for starting and warming up the engine.
Top right: Single lever outboard engine control with locking handle. The separate idling lever which also acts as choke, and an emergency stop switch is connected to the driver by the red spiral cord.
Bottom right: single lever control for side-mounting. It operates on the same principle as the twin-engine control.

Two-lever controls are almost pre-programmed for transmission damage. If you happen to get into a panic in a tricky situation, it's all too easy to forget about the throttle and consequently shift from 'full ahead' to 'full astern'.

This problem is not as serious with the single-lever control, where transmission and throttle are operated by the same lever. The path from ahead to astern – and vice versa – always goes through neutral (=engine idling). In this way gross mistakes in operation, to which beginners are particularly prone, can be substantially avoided. Single-lever controls all work on much the same principle, though there are numerous versions. Most models allow you to operate the throttle only, with the engine in neutral, for warming up or charging the batteries.

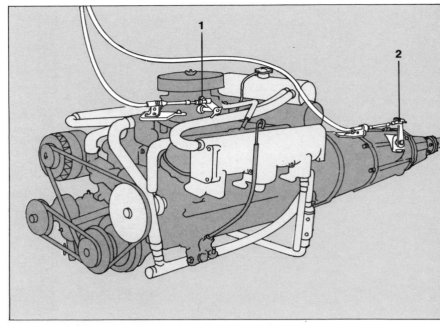

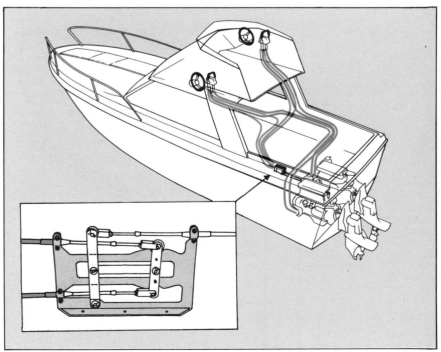

Top: Two teleflex cables control throttle and transmission (here a petrol engine driving a fixed shaft). Sometimes there's a third cable, for the petrol engine choke or the diesel stop button. Usually these are operated separately from the single lever control.

Below: Things get a bit more complicated where there are two helming positions. Transmission control (blue) is via a switch unit (inset). This transfers the activating movement from either helming position back to a single teleflex cable. Twin-engine installations (as shown here) need two switch units.

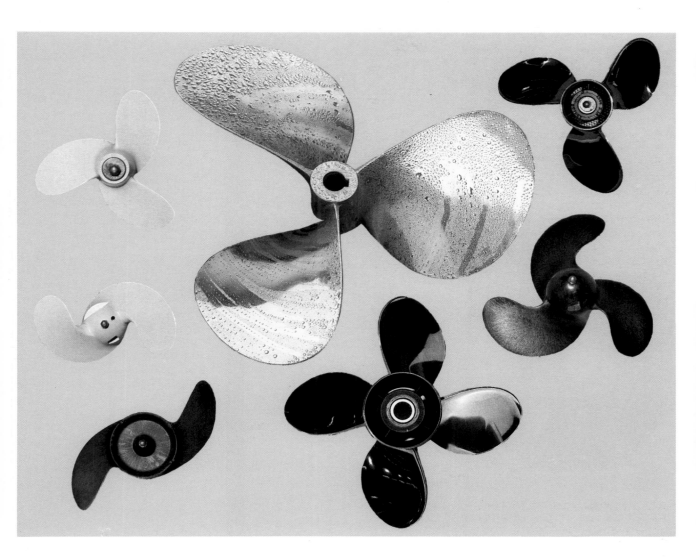

The driving force – the propeller

On the face of things, a propeller seems quite a simple component in a boat's transmission system – the last link in the chain which finally provides the thrust to drive the boat. Yet the propeller is probably the most complex and least understood part in the whole of a boat's power unit. It is often referred to as a 'screw', and yet the mechanical analogy is rather misleading. In fact, the propeller operates on the principle of a pump, drawing in water from one side, accelerating it, and ejecting it again on the other. The reaction this causes acts as a thrust on the propeller shaft, which causes the boat to move either forwards or astern. In a sense, therefore, the propeller is also a kind of jet-drive.

In motor-boating you will come across two, three and four-bladed propellers. The lightly loaded outboard propellers which drive fast planing craft are either two or three-

47

Right: Diameter, pitch and slip, shown for a 14 × 19 propeller: the theoretical pitch is 19 inches, the actual only 15 inches. The difference is slip, here 21%.

Below: Aluminium or steel propeller? The question to answer for outdrives, since props of both materials are usually available. Neither is faster than the other, even if that is sometimes promised. The steel prop is more robust but has a harsher take-up; aluminium is kinder to the transmission.

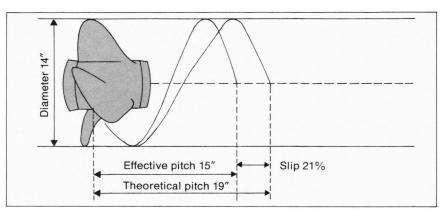

Effective pitch 15″ Slip 21%
Theoretical pitch 19″

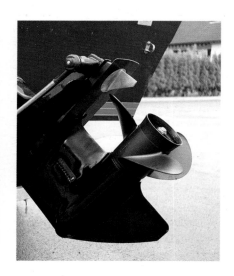

bladed, but those used by planing boats driven by fixed shafts or outdrives are usually three-bladed. Moderate sized displacement boats are generally fitted with three-bladed propellers, but larger, more powerful displacement boats – including many fishing and workboats – may have four-bladed props, which run more smoothly and can be more compact than three-bladed props of comparable thrust.

Diameter and pitch

Propeller size is specified by two measurements: diameter and pitch. These should be stamped into the propeller boss as two figures, the first referring to diameter and the second to pitch eg 15 × 19 (inches) or perhaps 330 × 530 (millimetres). The prop diameter is simply the diameter of the circle described by the propeller blades in one revolution, whereas pitch is measured according to the screw analogy and represents the distance forwards (or backwards) that the propeller would travel, in theory, in a solid medium – like a screw turning in wood.

Of course, water is not solid – it moves out of the way – and so a 15 × 19 inch propeller, following the screw analogy, would travel less than 19 inches in one revolution. There would be a certain amount of slip, the difference between the theoretical and actual advance of the propeller, which can vary between about 15 and 45% of pitch. Slip is often mistaken for inefficiency, and yet the two concepts – although closely related – are quite different. Slip is actually needed to

generate thrust from a propeller so, although slip is best kept fairly low, it's not a feature which you are trying to eliminate altogether. Because a propeller blade acts, to some extent, like the aerofoil of an aeroplane wing, without slip there would be no angle of attack between the propeller blade profile and the water current.

However, slip must remain within certain limits if the propeller is to operate efficiently. If there is too little slip, the engine will not attain its nominal revs; if there is too much, the propeller races without providing enough driving force. In both cases, efficiency is reduced and the scene is set for long-term engine wear. By following the screw analogy, you can calculate the theoretical speed of a boat from the pitch of its propeller and the engine revs. For example, our 15 × 19 inch prop turning at 2000 RPM would advance, if there were no slip, by:

19 × 2000 inches per minute
= 2 280 000 inches per hour
= 31.27 knots

If you know the slip, this has to be subtracted to find the actual speed; or, to put it another way, if the boat actually does 25 knots at 2000 RPM, then you know that the propeller slip is:

$$(31.27 - 25) \div 31.27 = 20\%.$$

Pitch is a critical factor when you are matching a propeller to a particular boat with a given engine horsepower. If the pitch is too low, the prop is effectively undergeared and the engine overrevs. If the pitch is too high, the propeller is overgeared for the speed the boat can realistically achieve or, to put it the other way round, the boat can't go as fast as the prop would like. In this case the engine will not reach its nominal revs.

With outboard motors and some outdrives, you can change propeller fairly easily and thereby match the pitch to your boat's load on a particular occasion. For example, if you were carrying six people and extra equipment aboard a small boat that usually carried two crew only, the engine would probably benefit from a slightly lower pitch and 'harder working' propeller.

The relationship between pitch and diameter is also important. Propellers for displacement craft are usually 'undersquare', which means that their pitch is less than the diameter. For example, a 6 ton motor yacht which cruises at 6 or 7 knots might have a 15 × 9 inch propeller. 'Oversquare' propellers (sometimes called speed props), where the pitch is greater than the diameter, are normally specified for all planing craft.

Propellers for outboards and outdrives are generally made of an aluminium-magnesium alloy, whose light weight is kinder on the small bevel gears used in the compact transmissions. Fixed shaft propellers used for heavier boats are invariably made of manganese bronze. Aluminium props are much more sensitive to impact than bronze props. Whereas a relatively slow turning bronze propeller might suffer a dent or a bent blade from hitting a piece of debris, the blade of an aluminium prop might well break off altogether.

Propeller problems

You can soon hear the effect of propeller problems. If a prop suddenly starts vibrating, you have probably picked up weed or a stray piece of rope or plastic. In such a situation, as indeed always if there is a suspicious change in the propeller noise, you need to throttle back and shift into neutral immediately.

Sometimes you can clear the problem by running astern briefly at idling revs, going into neutral again and letting the wind take the boat away a bit from the debris. Prop vibrations following a sharp blow can mean anything from a slight dent in one blade,

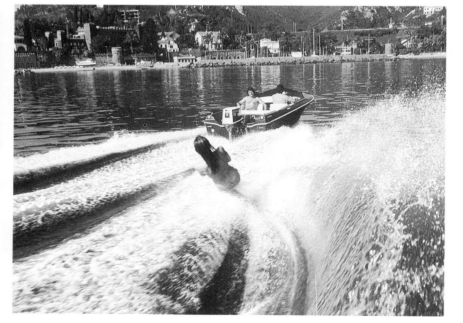

If you are keen on water-skiing, your standard prop probably won't do – you may need one with a lower pitch which, by virtue of higher engine revs, will produce the initial acceleration so important for easy starting on water-skis. Some engine manufacturers offer special water-ski props, but you will have to determine whether these are suitable for your own boat and engine.

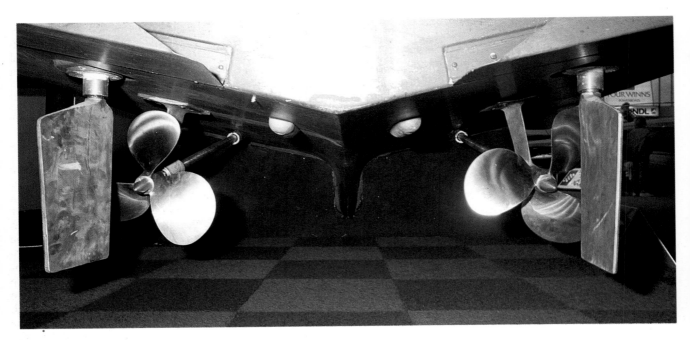

If you want vibration-free running, the clearance between the boat's bottom and the tip of the propellers should not be less than 10% of the prop diameter. Here the clearance is marginal.

with which you can run home quite safely, to a blade broken off or damage to the shaft or its bracket. In theory you must not carry on running with either of the latter two; in practice, however, there may be nothing else you can do. Very slowly, you make your way to the nearest boatyard or marina. Even a slightly bent blade should not be dismissed lightly as a 'cosmetic defect'. It has to be brought back to its proper pitch as soon as possible. If you don't do that, one blade provides more thrust than the other(s) and the shaft bracket is loaded unevenly. Something similar can happen if the leading edges have become notched. It's not enough just to have a go with a file, because that way you alter the blade widths. You then also get unbalanced centrifugal forces, because the blades no longer all have the same weight at the same distance from the centre of gravity.

The more serious these defects, the quicker the bearings will be ruined. In principle, hands off damaged props. Any DIY attempts with a file, emery paper or oilstone will only make things worse.

Highly irritating vibrations occur immediately if a fixed-shaft drive has the propeller too close to the bottom of the boat. This must be checked with the boat out of the water, and the blade tips should be at least 5% of the prop diameter clear of the bottom. But even then vibration can still occur; the normal clearance should be 10% of the diameter, and 12 to 15% is the ideal. A prop too close to the bottom may give rise to another dilemma: should its diameter turn out to be too small, nothing can be done about this other than by an expensive alteration of the whole engine installation involving a more steeply inclined prop shaft.

What is cavitation?

Cavitation is an apparently mysterious process which propeller experts like to introduce into the conversation with bit of a frown. Cavitation is another way of saying 'a formation of vapour bubbles at the propeller with destructive effect'. Because the accelerated water on the leading face of the blade flows very fast, a depression is set up there and the water begins to 'boil', forming bubbles of vapour. These effectively 'thicken' the blades, increasing their resistance to rotation through the water and lowering the propeller output. Over the trailing face of the blade the flow slows down again, causing a steep increase in pressure with the result that when they get there the bubbles collapse again abruptly – with the speed of sound. They strike the metal so sharply that they can literally knock holes in it.

Such cavitation can occur if a boat, too heavy for its engines, is laboriously forced along at full power. It can also be caused by a ragged blade leading edge, too great a curvature of the blade, or a rough blade surface. Cavitating propellers can be recognised by curious humming and rumbling noises. If a prop in normal operation shows the erosion of the back (pressure) faces of the blades typical of cavitation, only a specialist workshop can help – you hope. Usually the very design of the boat is at the root of the trouble, by, for example, allowing the prop to draw air down from the surface so that it is continuously churning around in an air-water mixture less dense than solid water.

Right-handed and turning clockwise are not the same thing

If, with the boat driving ahead, a propeller turns to the right, ie clockwise, seen from astern, it is said to be right-handed. Conversely, a prop turning to the left with the boat driving ahead is left-handed. Since when going astern the direction of rotation of propellers is reversed, a right-handed one then turns to the left and a left-handed one to the right. In other words: this prop now turning to the right remains left-handed. Or: right-handed and turning to the right are not the same thing, but are often confused. Most single-screw motor boats have right-handed propellers. Motor yachts with twin engines usually have a left-handed one on the left (port) side and a right-handed one on the right (starboard) side. These are called outwards-turning propellers. Rarer are inwards-turning ones, with a right-handed prop on the left and a left-handed prop on the right. Comparisons have shown that whether propellers are in- or outwards turning makes no significant difference to efficiency and operating characteristics, or to a boat's manoeuvring qualities.

The paddlewheel effect

Propellers don't just produce drive forwards or astern. There is usually a marked sideways thrust which, with single-engine boats, can either help or hinder manoeuvring in confined spaces. This effect is caused by the propeller acting partly as a paddlewheel *across* the boat. Now you might think that such a paddle could only be effective if the top half was out of the water; with the prop fully immersed, surely any sideways drive produced by the 'bottom' blades would be cancelled out by sideways drive in the opposite direction produced by the 'top' blades? However, the paddlewheel thrust from the bottom of the propeller is actually more effective than that from the top, since the lower half of the prop acts in slightly deeper

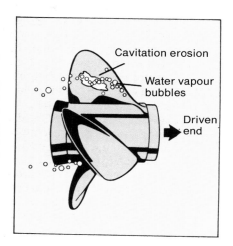

Cavitation erosion

Water vapour bubbles

Driven end

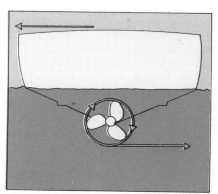

The paddlewheel effect with a right-handed prop, the stern kicks to port when you go astern.

water and is less prone to the turbulence which occurs near the surface. Therefore, the bottom blades usually win the battle of the sideways thrust and a right-handed propeller will tend to swing the stern to starboard when driving ahead and to port when driving astern.

Twin-engine boats usually have opposite-handed propellers fitted, so that the two paddlewheel effects cancel each other out. However, you will certainly notice a significant sideways thrust if one engine is out of action and you are trying to manoeuvre with the remaining engine. With single outboard or outdrive, you can often neutralise any paddlewheel effect by adjusting the trim tab underneath the cavitation plate.

The Duoprop

Just when everyone thought that propellers had reached the end of their development, the Swedish engine builders Volvo Penta came up with a cunning invention which they called 'Duoprop'. Two contra-rotating propellers sit one behind the other on one shaft; the first on a hollow length into which the solid shaft for the second fits. The trick is that the propulsive column of water accelerated by the first propeller is so-to-speak 'tailored' to fit the second. By this means the high-loss twist normally given to the wake is converted into a straight flow which significantly reinforces the propeller thrust. The result is reduced consumption and increased maximum speed. This is the point to introduce the terms 'brake horsepower' and 'shaft horsepower', being closely connected with propeller and trans-

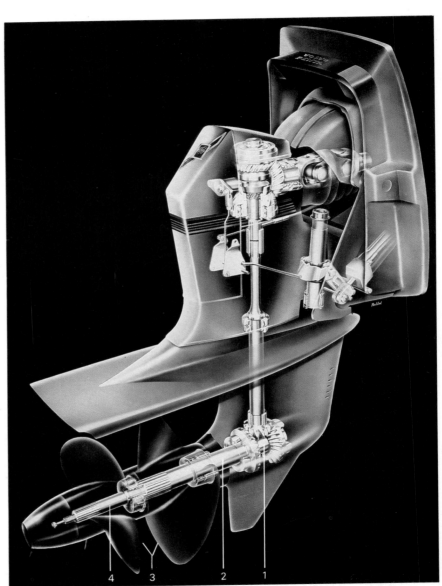

The efficient Duoprop is often installed on outdrives and outboards. The final transmission is slightly modified with this system.
1 The bottom bevel gear operates as it would for a single prop.
2 The inner (forward) prop turns on a hollow outer shaft.

3 Three-bladed propellers are normally used with a fast-revving petrol engine. Slower running diesels use a three-bladed outer prop and a four-bladed inner.
4 A contra-rotating inner shaft carries the outer (aft) propeller.

mission efficiency. Brake horsepower (BHP) is the maximum horsepower developed by an engine at a given rpm, as tested by the engine manufacturer. Shaft horsepower (SHP) is power actually transmitted to the propeller at a given rpm.

To estimate shaft horsepower, engineers usually work on about 3% of brake horsepower being lost in the gearbox and a further 1½% lost to the friction of each propeller shaft bearing. That doesn't sound too bad, but it's also interesting to see how efficiently, overall, an engine converts the chemical energy from its fuel into power to turn the propeller. As a rough average, you can reckon that about 35% of energy is lost as heat to the atmosphere, 25% as heat and vibration to the water and a net 2% is lost at the prop shaft. This only leaves about 38% of the energy in the fuel for propulsion. Of this 38%, about 65% is actually converted into forward thrust by the propeller and 35% is lost in turning the propeller itself.

This 65% of available shaft horsepower converted into thrust to drive

the boat is known as propeller efficiency. The Duoprop is able to increase this efficiency to something like 75% which results, not only in the boat going faster, but also in a fuel saving of about 15%.

The steering wheel aboard a boat seems, in appearance rather like that of a car, but the similarity ends there. It's true that to change direction you also turn the wheel the same way, although when you are steering a boat

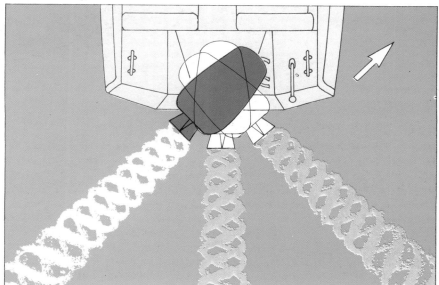

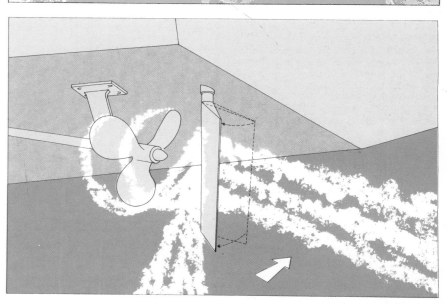

Top right: *Steering with outboards and outdrives:* Angle the drive towards the left and the prop thrust pushes the stern to the right (starboard). When going astern, angling to the left causes the prop to *pull* the stern to the left (port). The effective use of the prop thrust makes very tight turns possible.

Right: *Fixed-shaft drive with rudder:* The rudder blade is inclined to the flow produced by the propeller, which is directed straight astern. Impact pressure is applied to the blade, pushing the stern in the required direction. However the steering effect is nothing like as pronounced as with a steering prop, so the turning circle is roughly twice as great.

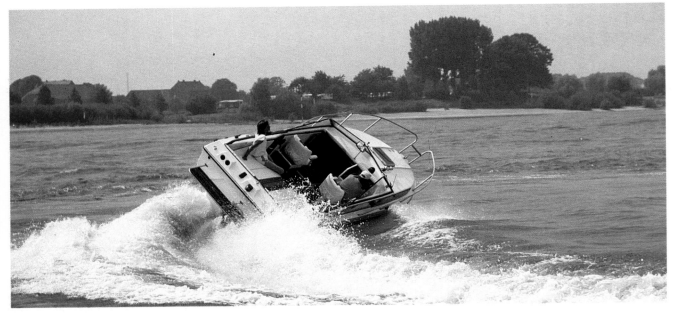

A really tight turn, possible only with a steering prop.

with a tiller, or steering an outboard by hand, you move the tiller to the right to steer to the left and vice versa.

Boats with outboards or outdrives are steered by swivelling the entire engine/hinged part of the drive. That diverts the propeller wake, the direction of prop thrust. The stern moves the way it is pushed by the prop going ahead, or pulled when going astern.

As a result these boats have a very small turning circle and are splendidly manoeuvrable in a restricted space. They don't have a rudder, though, and that does have its disadvantages. The slower you are moving, the less the steerability. Indeed, with the engine in neutral you lose steering altogether because the shaft unit itself has only a minimal rudder effect.

With fixed shaft drives steering is effected by turning the rudder blade behind the propeller. The pressure of the propeller wake on the rudder blade pushes the stern in the opposite direction. However, because only a part of the wake can be used to obtain this result (part of it is beyond the rudder's reach) the effect is less powerful than with a steerable propeller. When going astern, the propeller wake is directed ahead. The rudder is then in a suction zone and responds only to the speed of the boat through the water. The rudder effect in reverse is accordingly poor, particularly if the prop shaft comes through the bottom at an especially steep angle, ie is inclined downwards strongly. But with a rudder blade, you do have steerage way as long as the boat is moving through the water – even with the engine out of gear.

Typical steering systems for boats with outboards use a car-type steering wheel and a cable reel for the operating cable. Fixed rack and pinion steering is sometimes found in boats with inboard engines, but a system of rotating rods and universal joints is more common.

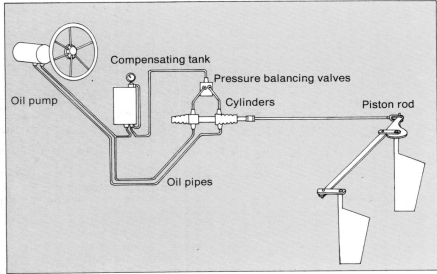

Hydraulic steering gear: Comfortable steering for larger yachts.

The mitigated risk – the fuel tank and system

You would think you could rely on the fuel tanks and systems which yards fit into their boats, and most of the time that faith would be justified. But not always! So it's a good idea to know one's way reasonably well round this aspect of an engine installation. Since any petrol leaking out combines with air to form an explosive mixture, boats with petrol engines have particularly severe safety requirements for these systems.

The tank should be in a space sealed off by a bulkhead, so that in the event of the tank leaking the fuel does not spread through the whole boat. This requirement is flouted more often than one would imagine. Although leaking diesel tanks don't immediately conjure up thoughts of the fearful danger of an explosion, diesel leaks do create a horrible mess in the bilges. The tank should be installed so

securely that it can't be torn loose by the violent motion which is typical of fast planing craft. There must be a shut-off tap at the tank, not just somewhere along the line – otherwise a break in the line might let fuel run into the bilge. For safety's sake that tap should be shut whenever the boat is not running, especially with petrol engines. Between the tank and the engine(s) you should fit a large capacity water separator and then an in-line renewable-cartridge fuel filter. These should be duplicated if you have twin engines.

Not quite the same are the so-called agglomerators, a combination of filter and separator. These won't do for larger diesel engines; they need a proper heavy-duty separator. If there isn't one – and that's not infrequent – you should have one fitted. Best of all, fit two filter systems in parallel, with a

changeover valve for switching from one to the other. If the filter in use becomes choked, (the engine begins to stutter) because the movement of the boat has stirred up dirt in the tank, you can switch over to the other; that's quicker than changing a filter cartridge in a boat rolling in a seaway. Frequently, the filters are fixed to the engine, simply because its easier to mount them there. This is not a good idea because stirred-up dirt from the tank can then clog the whole length of the fuel supply line.

Fuel system for a diesel: In principle, the tank installations for a diesel are broadly similar to petrol engines from the filler to the supply pump. The petrol engine has a carburettor in lieu of the injection pump. Diesels have a fuel return line, for taking fuel surplus to the injectors' requirements back to the tank. In some cases it's taken back only as far as the supply pump.

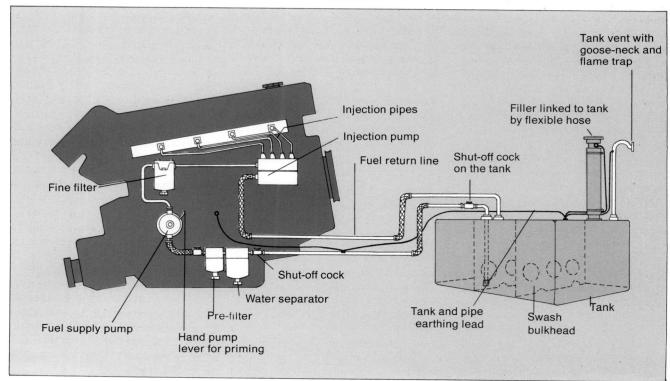

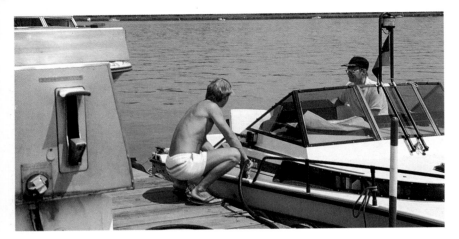

The filling pipe must make a gas-tight joint with the tank and must extend nearly to its bottom. That prevents any static electricity spark which might be generated at the filler aperture when fuelling, from penetrating into the tank. At the filler hole on deck, the pipe must have a large, tight-fitting collar so that neither fuel nor vapour can get into the boat through the gap between the pipe and the edge of the hole in the deck. To stop the fuel 'hiccuping' during fuelling and squirting overboard to contaminate the environment, the bore of the filling pipe should be at least 38 mm (1½ in). If that minimum requirement has not been met, fuelling becomes a very delicate operation. The tank vent allows the vapour in the tank to escape when fuelling. To ensure its unimpeded flow, a vent pipe bore of at least 13 mm (½ in) is necessary. The vent also serves as an overflow pipe, and must be led outboard through a gas-tight opening in the boat's side so that any vapour discharge or fuel overflowing can only escape on to the water and not find its way into the bilge. The opening through the hull must have a flame trap. The whole installation, including the filling connection, must be earthed.

Plain mild steel may be used as material for petrol tanks, but it should be galvanised. Better, and more expensive, are tanks made of Monel metal,

stainless steel or seawater proof aluminium alloy. For diesel fuel tanks, structural steel or self-quenching synthetic resin are suitable materials. Copper alloys such as Monel metal and also steel galvanised on the inside are suitable for diesel tanks.

Tanks of more than 50 litre capacity, which in practice includes all motor boat tanks, should be subdivided by baffle bulkheads to prevent fuel sloshing about. Large quantities of fuel on the move put a strain on tank mountings and can possibly impair the stability of the boat and threaten its safety. Diesel tanks must never be sucked entirely dry, because the pumps will suck in air which can stop the engine dead. Bleeding air out of the system again is time-consuming and, in a seaway with the boat rolling, not without its problems.

The business of fuelling

According to statistics, most accidents involving an explosion and subsequent fire happen immediately after fuelling because an ignitable petrol-air mixture has formed in the boat. The igniting spark may then come from switching on the ignition, from a loose, defective, electric cable shorting to earth, or from an unscreened generator which it is still entirely possible

to find aboard motor boats. So when you are fuelling there are precautions which substantially reduce the risks, though with petrol engines danger can never be entirely eliminated.

Before fuelling:
- If possible moor the boat so that the wind comes from ahead.
- Stop the engine, no smoking, all open flames extinguished (cooker, gas refrigerator).
- Windows and scuttles closed tight.

During fuelling:
- Establish metal-to-metal contact between fuel nozzle and filling connection before letting fuel flow, because frequently there is a difference of electric potential between the boat and the shore which can lead to the generation of sparks.
- Don't operate any electric switches.
- Don't step ashore from the boat, or on board from the shore.

When fuelling is over, open all windows and scuttles again to ensure thorough ventilation of the compartments. Before starting the engine, the blower (ventilating fan) in the engine compartment should be run for about four minutes. You have to be patient before casting off. Indeed, running the blower every time before starting the engine should be a cast-iron rule, to draw off any petrol vapour in the bilge, even if only in a weak concentration. But how often do you see the blower not being switched on at all, or the engine being started after it has only run for a few seconds? With such carelessness in mind, some boat builders have combined the ignition switch with the blower circuit. When you switch on initially, only the blower starts.

On-board electrics

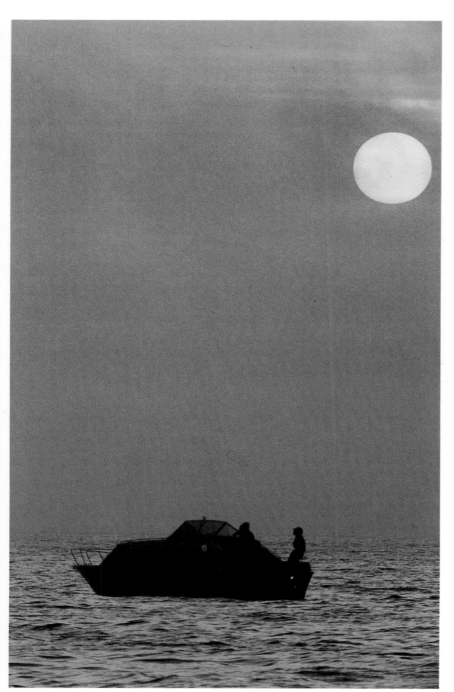

Aboard small runabouts and sports boats, electrics might only be used to start the engine and perhaps run the navigation lights, an echo-sounder or a VHF radio. Aboard modern motor cruisers, however, the electrical systems are often more sophisticated than you have at home. Even a modest seagoing motor yacht would probably be running a wide range of electrical equipment which could include cabin lighting, navigation and deck lights, an electric bilge pump, anchor winch; navigation equipment such as Decca, Loran and radar; a VHF radio, an autopilot, refrigerator, central heating, engine room fans ... the list goes on and on.

To supply all this auxiliary equipment as well as start one or two large engines, you need two batteries or banks of batteries, each with its own separate circuit. It is important to keep the engine starting battery for that purpose alone, so that it's always fully topped-up and ready for action, even if all the ship's domestic equipment has been heavily used.

The batteries used aboard boats are usually heavy-duty lead-acid 12 volt accumulators of much greater capacity than you'd find in your car. Larger yachts sometimes use banks of 12 volt batteries connected in parallel to provide a more efficient 24 volt system. The capacity of an accumulator is rated in ampere-hours (Ah). For starting outboards up to about 100 hp and running a basic set of navigation lights, you can get by with one 60 Ah battery. But once you have to start a fairly large diesel engine and run even a few items of domestic and navigation equipment, you will need two batteries of about 120 Ah each.

Ideally, the starter battery should be of a type designed for high loads of short duration. It is normally wired to

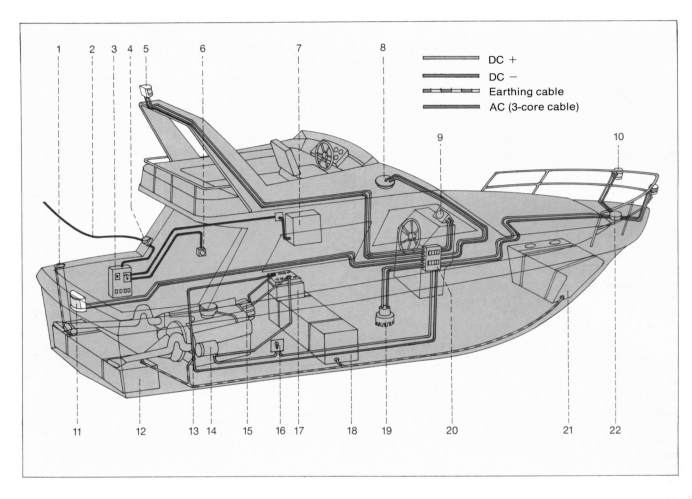

A schematic wiring plan for AC and DC. Always go by the colours: Brown is used for the supply leads (+); light blue for the return or neutral leads (−) which are also earthing leads in a DC circuit (in older boats you can still find red for + ve and black for − ve). Green/yellow cables link all major metal parts such as tanks, tank filler inlet stub(s), and engine. They don't have any electrical supply function but are important for safety, forming an earth whch keeps all metal parts at the same potential and so prevents any static charge building up. This not only prevents galvanic corrosion and interference with electronic instruments, but

also avoids the risk of a petrol-air mixture explosion, which could be caused by an electric spark when fuelling.

1   Fuel filler
2. Shorepower cable
3   AC circuit breaker
4   Shore connection socket
5   Steaming light
6   AC socket
7   AC load
8   Internal lighting
9   Helming position instruments (the same supply and return lines of

course go also to the second position on the flybridge, but these have been omitted for clarity)
10   Sidelights
11   Stern light
12   Fuel tank
13   Earthing connection
14   Starter
15   Lighting generator
16   Main breaker
17   Battery(ies)
18   Sewerage tank
19   Bilge pump
20   DC distribution panel
21   Fresh water tank
22   Junction box

supply the engine monitoring instruments. The auxiliary battery (or batteries) should be of a high capacity, with thicker plates suitable for long duration discharge. The auxiliary circuit supplies all other loads and the two circuits are only connected via the charging system of the engine. With two batteries it is important to have a heavy-duty changeover switch, so that if necessary you can start the engine using the general purpose battery.

Power consumption

Whether you are running a small motor cruiser or a large yacht, it is important to have a clear picture of the energy requirements of all your electrical equipment and to arrange the capacity of the batteries so that they can supply all the power that is needed. Yachtsmen are often surprised when they tot up the consumption of all their lights, pumps, navigation electronics, and any domestic equipment such as fridges.

As the capacity of a battery is measured in ampere-hours (Ah), therefore a 90 Ah battery in prime condition should be able to supply a current of 10 amps for 9 hours or 5 amps for 18 hours. In other words:

Current requirement (Amps) × Operating time (hours) = Necesssary battery capacity (Ah).

It is well worth adding up the likely and maximum consumption for your own boat, to check whether your auxiliary batteries are large enough to cope. If you don't know the actual current taken by an item of equipment, you can calculate this from the relation:

Consumption table for:

1 Day-cruiser (about 7 metres) Navigation lights	Output (Watts)	Current (amps) 12 V	24 V
Side lights	25	2.08	1.04
Stern light	10	0.83	0.42
Steaming light	25	2.08	1.04
Anchor light (all-round)	25	2.08	1.04
Internal lighting	150	12.5	6.25
Instrument illumination	10	0.83	0.42
Echo sounder	2	0.17	0.09
Log/speedo	1	0.08	0.04
Bilge pump	100	8.33	4.17
2 Motor yacht (about 12 metres) (additional)			
Radar	60	5.00	2.5
Decca or Loran C	2	0.17	0.09
Compass repeater	10	0.83	0.42
Autopilot	20	1.67	0.84
Signal hooter/siren	100	8.33	4.17
Searchlight	150	12.50	6.25
Clear-view screen	50	4.17	2.09
Anchor winch	1200	100.00	50.00
Fresh water pump	100	8.33	4.17
3-plate cooker + oven*	3000		
Refrigerator	80	6.67	3.34
Heating**	150	12.50	6.25
Water heater*	1000...5000		
Electric WC	80	6.67	3.34
Ventilating fans	100	8.33	4.17
Engine compartment blower	100	8.33	4.17
Gas detector	5	0.42	0.21
Σ			

*Only for connection to 240 V
**Starting load

$$\text{Current consumption (Amps)} = \frac{\text{Power rating (Watts)}}{\text{Voltage (Volts)}}$$

An 8 watt fluorescent light, for example, powered from a 12 volt supply uses $\frac{8}{12} = \frac{2}{3}$ amp of current.

The table on page 59 gives an estimate of the current requirements of the most common items of boat electrical equipment. You can pick out your own loads from this table and draw up a power inventory list. This will give you a good idea of the battery capacity required for your boat.

You have to distinguish between those loads which are only switched on when the engine is running and those which are fed entirely by the ship's battery when the engine is stopped. Navigation equipment comes into the first group, but the internal lighting, the refrigerator, heating equipment and the anchor light fall into the second. When including these latter items in the calculation it pays to be generous.

A further distinction when assessing power requirements is between short and long duration loads. The former include, for example, the signal horn, searchlight, engine compartment blower, and even the WC. The anchor winch may take 100 amps at 12 volts or 50 amps at 24 volts, and yet will operate only for minutes at a time usually when the engine or generator is running. A much more significant drain will be caused by two bright cabin lights left on for most of an evening.

Having worked out your theoretical power requirements, you need to bear in mind that batteries give less voltage as they become discharged and it is not realistic to expect a 90 Ah battery to supply 9 amps for a full 10

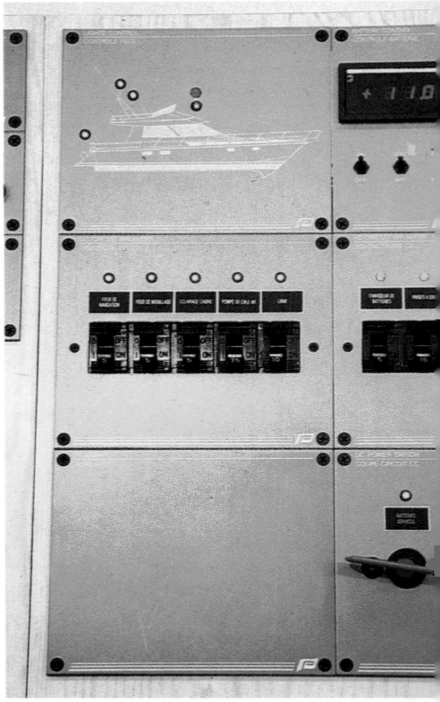

Switchboard with space for expansion, which comprises several smaller panels and may be enlarged as required. Top left: the navigation light monitor with current-indicating LEDs. Alongside: a digital multi-purpose indicator, usable as a voltmeter and ammeter, switchable to No 1 or No 2 battery. Underneath, the 240V AC distributor with automatic cut-outs for battery charger and plug sockets. On the left of that, automatic cut-outs for the various loads in the boat's DC system. Bottom right: the battery main breaker. A good and sensible arrangement.

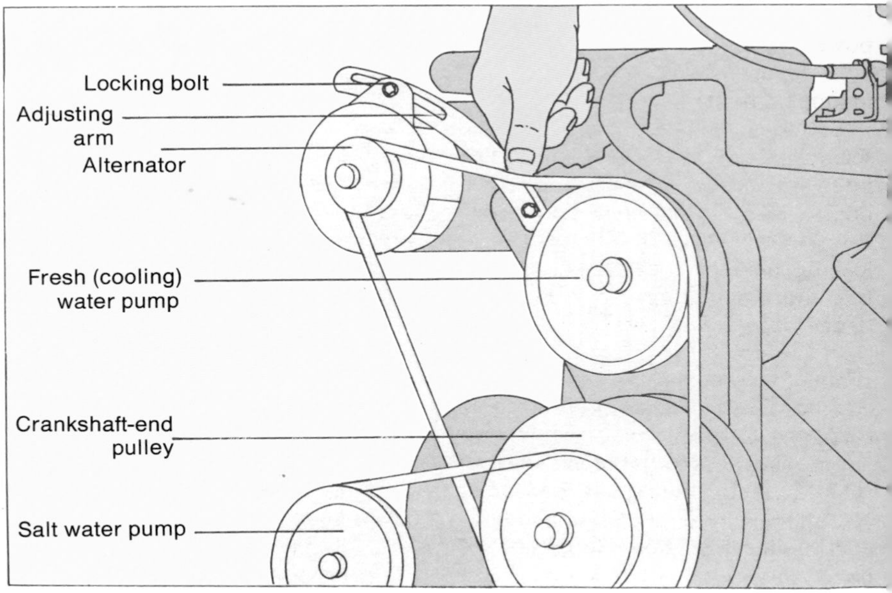
Locking bolt
Adjusting arm
Alternator
Fresh (cooling) water pump
Crankshaft-end pulley
Salt water pump

The thumb-pressure test: You should be able to push the V-belt down a good 8 mm. The tension is adjusted using the arm connected to the alternator.

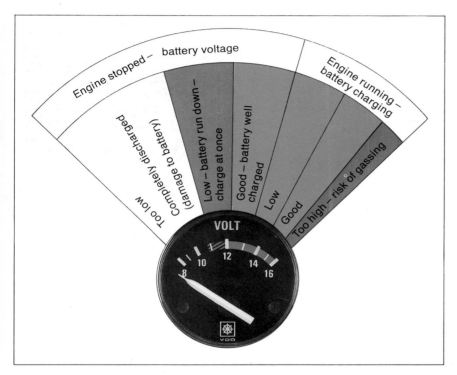

Engine stopped – battery voltage

Engine running – battery charging

Too low

Completely discharged (damage to battery)

Low – battery run down – charge at once

Good – battery well charged

Low

Good

Too high – risk of gassing

VOLT

8   10   12   14   16

VDO

Left: *Voltmeter*: With an 8 to 16 V scale for a 12V installation (18 to 32 for 24 V), which allows you to monitor the state of charge of the battery. At the 'rest potential' – reached about an hour after applying load – the voltmeter pretty accurately indicates the battery's state of charge, based on the acid density. At 12.7 V it is fully charged, at 11.6 V run down. At 10.5 V it is totally discharged and on the way out. A battery at anything below 12 V has to be charged. The charging potential lies between 14 and 14.4 V. Above that, the battery starts gassing, which is bad for it, and indicates that the voltage control is defective.

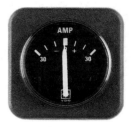

AMP

30   – +   30

Above: *Ammeter*: shows whether the alternator is charging properly (+), or whether too many loads are draining the battery (–).

hours. You need to multiply your total power requirements by 1.5 to 2 to calculate a safe working battery capacity in ampere hours.

Batteries should be installed securely. This is something you absolutely must check in the case of a new boat – that the batteries cannot fall over or break loose. Not only does leaking acid corrode metal objects, but short circuiting can also cause dangerous arcing and thus easily starts fires. Ideally, the batteries should be 'non-spill' – the kind that can be tilted or overturned without acid running out.

Nickel-cadmium batteries have certain advantages aboard a boat. The NiCad battery can safely withstand overloading, complete discharge and heavy shocks. It has a long life – ten

years or more, compared with three or four years for the usual lead storage battery. The disadvantages of NiCad batteries are their weight and greater initial cost.

Boat batteries are normally recharged by one or more alternators driven by the engine via a V-belt. Silicon diode rectifiers convert the alternating current into the required 12 volt or 24 volt direct current which a central switchboard distributes to the individual loads. Each circuit should be protected by a fuse or an automatic circuit breaker. A good insight into the quality of workmanship aboard a boat is obtained by inspecting the electrical distribution box. If a hopeless tangle of wires jumps out at you, be prepared for trouble.

The alternator V-belt is correctly

tensioned if it can be flexed about 8 mm by thumb pressure. The belt tension should be checked about every 50 running hours. If it is too tight, the alternator bearings will wear rapidly. If the belt is too loose, the alternator's revs will be too low and its charging rate reduced; the belt itself will also wear much more quickly.

Most larger cruising yachts have a second electrical circuit for 240 volt AC mains, which is supplied via a shore connection whilst in harbour. At the distribution point, the AC switchboard, it is vital to have a circuit breaker or heavy duty fuse to protect against overload. Having a mains circuit on board is very convenient because it allows you to use almost any item of electrical household equipment.

Where, as is often the case with motor yachts, engine running times are relatively short, the amount of charging supplied by the main engine(s) may not suffice for a high power requirement. In this case an auxiliary generator is a must, one that is entirely independent of the main engine generator and shore connection, and feeds 12 volt/24 volt DC or 240 volt AC directly into the relevant circuit. An auxiliary generator may be of the lightweight portable type or installed permanently on board. More sophisticated two-way charger converters are sometimes used on boats to step-up and convert 12 or 24 volt DC well as acting as standard chargers which are able to convert mains shore power into DC to charge the batteries directly.

Batteries discharge themselves slowly over long periods. In Mediterranean summer temperatures, this can happen at a rate of several percent of capacity per day. So even if your batteries are fully charged when you leave the boat, some of that charge will have been lost by the time you come on board again. It is therefore important to have good battery instruments, so that you can quickly assess the state of all your batteries on board.

The voltmeter – sometimes called a battery state meter – shows the actual voltage across the battery terminals. For a nominal 12 volt battery, this voltage can vary from about 11 to 11.5 volts, when the battery is well down, to 13 volts when the battery is fully charged. When the engine is running, the voltmeter will show the voltage generated by the alternator, normally somewhere between 13 and 15 volts with everything working properly.

The ammeter shows the amount of charging current going into the batteries, or the discharge from them. When the batteries are well down, the charging current will be high, but this steadily reduces towards zero as the batteries become topped up.

Signpost at sea – the compass

For river and estuary sailors a compass is not an absolute requirement, but as soon as you start boating in coastal waters the compass becomes an indispensable 'pathfinder' in the uncertain vastness of the open sea. Even if you intend to remain in sight of familiar reference points, adverse circumstances such as fog suddenly rolling in or darkness falling before you get home can quickly deprive you of your sense of direction. A compass is an extremely sensitive instrument, liable to be influenced by any iron or steel components on board, the fields of cables permanently or temporarily carrying current, or the permanent magnets in motors, loudspeakers and other appliances. For that reason a compass should be installed as far as possible from any of these items, ideally at least two metres from engines and autopilot switching relays, one metre from radar or radio telephone sets, windscreen wiper motors and loudspeakers, and 0.6 metres from all engine-monitoring instruments and anything made of iron. In some boats, especially those built of steel, minimum distances cannot easily be maintained in any

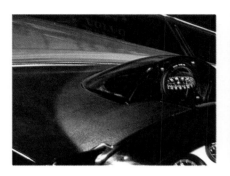

well-equipped helming position if the helmsman is to be able to read the compass easily. In this case a repeater compass is often used, with the master unit installed in a magnetically neutral position and the repeater, which is nothing more than a remote indicator, mounted near the helm position. An example of such a repeater is shown in the photograph below.

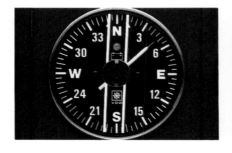

The cockpit instrumentation – and what it reveals

To a large extent, the selection of instruments and navigational equipment is a very personal affair. Some boat owners like to keep things simple, while others prefer to see an array of meters and displays which make you think more of an aircraft's cockpit than a boat. Much also depends on the type and size of the vessel.

A small runabout may have little more than a rev counter and an oil pressure warning light, but the instrumentation for a twin-engined motor yacht with turbo chargers and charge cooling can soon add up to twenty or so indicators.

While some navigation equipment might be said to fall under the heading of 'gadgets', any instruments which accurately monitor the wellbeing of the engine(s) contribute significantly to safety and earn their place aboard a seagoing boat.

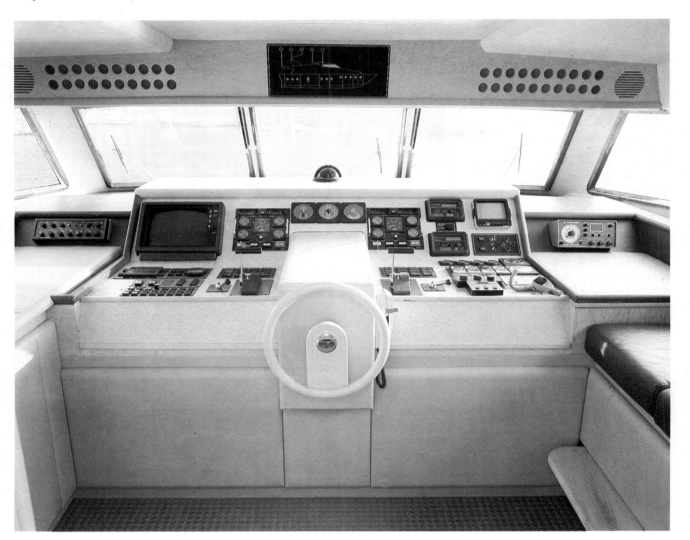

Oil pressure gauge   Oil temperature gauge   Cooling water
                                               temperature gauge

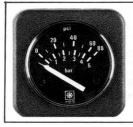 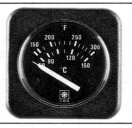 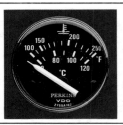

Let us therefore take a look at a well-instrumented helming position:

Oil pressure gauge In the case of diesels and four-stroke petrol engines, a gearwheel pump feeds oil from the sump to the big-end bearings, shafts and all other important moving parts. This system of lubrication calls for a relatively constant oil pressure, between 3 bar and 6 bar for most engines. The simplest device for monitoring the lubricating circuit is an oil pressure warning light. This lights up when the ignition key is turned to 'run' and goes out as soon as the engine is running and has built up oil pressure. It lights up again if for any reason the oil pressure drops. A meter that gives an actual reading of the oil pressure provides you with even more information about how well the system is working.

A separate transmission oil gauge is needed for hydraulically controlled transmissions. It quickly shows up any loss of oil which could otherwise result in damage to, or even failure of, the transmission.

Oil temperature gauge Since the lubricating oil also helps to cool the engine, particularly the bearings, there needs to be a reservoir of oil which the oil pump can draw on and which is allowed to cool for a while before it is circulated again. For smallish engines, measuring the oil pressure suffices, but not if engine and/or transmission are fitted with an oil cooler. The oil temperature gauge indicates when the engine has warmed sufficiently to be ready for full load. Sustained high revs at temperatures below 60°C can cause engine damage. Temperatures above 120°C indicate damaged bearings, incorrect ignition setting or cooling water shortage.

Cooling water temperature gauge To produce a rapid rise in cooling water temperature on starting, and maintain a steady favourable operating temperature, there is a thermostatic control valve in the cooling water circuit. The normal optimum operating temperature lies somewhere between 70° and 100°C, depending on the engine. Irregularities in the cooling system, whether due to insufficient tension in the V-belt driving the pump, deposits on the cooling surfaces or clogged sea water valves, will in a very short time cause serious damage to the engine. So the temperature gauge is an indispensable, basic, instrument.

Cooling water pressure gauge The water required for cooling is normally pumped through the system with a pressure of at least 1 bar. A significant drop in that pressure indicates defects in the cooling system.

Fuel pressure gauge The fuel supply pump of diesels and petrol engines

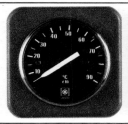 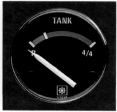 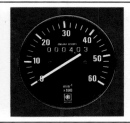 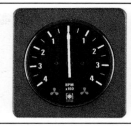 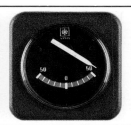

produces a pressure of about 0.6 bar. Too low a pressure may indicate air in the fuel, a leak in the line, a defective pump or a dirty fuel filter.

Tank contents gauge (Fuel or water). This is particularly important for inaccessible and triangular tanks, where checking by dipstick is really not practicable.

Exhaust temperature gauge For diesel engines, level exhaust temperatures indicate an even loading of all cylinders; in addition, the temperature itself is a measure of the engine load. It normally has a certain value for any given rev range; at full power around 600°C. Deviations are an indication of dirty filters or some other defect.

Charge pressure gauge The output of engines fitted with turbochargers depends on charge pressure. If this is less than 1 bar there is usually something wrong with the engine or the turbocharging system and the engine must not then be run at more than half power.

Monitoring the battery The minimum indicator requirement is a charging warning light. Like the oil pressure indicator, this will light up when the ignition key is turned to 'run'. It goes out as soon as the engine is running and the alternator voltage exceeds that of the battery. If the warning light

remains on or starts to flicker whilst under way, either the V-belt driving the generator is too loose or there is some other defect. The two warning lights come on again when the engine is switched off, because the alternator stops charging and the oil pressure drops. The voltmeter and ammeter were dealt with on page 62.

Engine hour meter All maintenance intervals are given in engine running hours. Without an engine hour meter there is no hope of sticking to the maintenance programme accurately, and yet such maintenance is particularly important for boat engines whose running is much interrupted. Engine hour meters can also be used for measuring fuel consumption provided you know what the hourly consumption is at certain revs.

Rev-differential meters Useful instruments for twin-engined boats. If the revs on each engine differ markedly, irritating vibrations are set up and the boat no longer runs straight, which has to be compensated for by applying rudder. This causes increased resistance which means higher fuel consumption. Because of certain installation-dependent tolerances, separate rev counters may not indicate such differences clearly enough, whereas rev-differential metres allow you to match the revs of both engines more accurately.

Rudder angle indicator Useful for all manoeuvres in restricted spaces, where repeated backing and filling quickly cause you to lose the feel for the position of the rudder. Particularly handy in boats with outdrives, whose propellers themselves, rather than a rudder, steer the boat. Also indispensable in yachts with hydraulic steering gear. In larger vessels, the rudder position indicator often gives the first indication that you are being set off from your direct course by a cross-current. When you are steering visually, the rudder angle tells you approximately how many degrees you have to hold up.

Trim angle indicator Permits precise matching of the trim tab setting to different speeds and loadings of the boat.

Fuel flow meter Indicates present consumption for petrol engines in ℓ/h (no use for diesels and engines with fuel return systems). Used in conjunction with log and rev counter on trial runs, it allows you to draw up a curve or table of ranges at various speeds, and shows at what revs and speed the boat will be running most economically. Increased fuel consumption for no obvious reason can be an alarm signal.

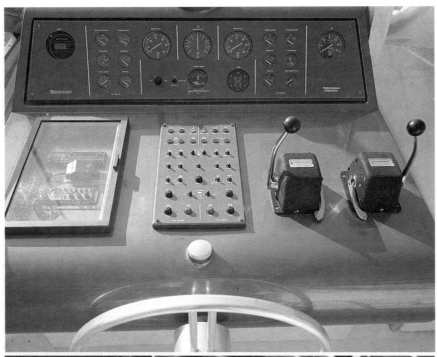

The helming position of a 24.5 metre yacht with twin engines of 2100 hp. All instruments, in a console arranged to avoid dazzle, are fully in the field of vision. Starting top left: digital echo sounder – voltmeter 1 – water temperature gauge 1 – rev counter 1 – rev differential meter – rev counter 2 – water temperature gauge 2 – voltmeter 2 – log. Middle row, from the left: Engine hour meter 1 – oil pressure gauge 1 – oil pressure gauge 2 – Engine hour meter 2. Bottom row, from left: engine compartment temperature gauge – transmission oil pressure gauge 1 – rudder angle indicator – trim tab angle indicator – transmission oil pressure gauge 2 – sea water temperature gauge. On the left in the desk (with cover): marine radio and satellite navigation system. Alongside, start and stop buttons for the diesels, operational indicator and warning lights, and switches for all important auxiliary equipment.

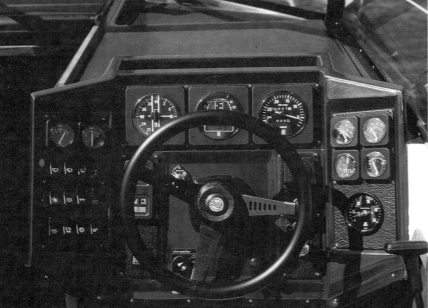

The practical curved instrument console of an 8.8 metre motor cruiser with 1 × 192 hp: left side: voltmeter, ammeter. Underneath, ready to hand, the switches for windscreen wipers, anchor winch, navigation lights, internal lighting, anchor light, bilge pump, blower, etc. Above the steering wheel the heading indicator of a remote compass system, alongside this the echo sounder (the associated alarm on the left, half hidden by the wheel) and log. On the right side: water temperature and oil pressure. Underneath: Engine hour meter, tank level indicator, rev counter. On the left behind the steering wheel, at the top the trim tab switch, at the bottom the heating. On the right, hidden by the wheel, audible warning device, horn and ignition lock.

Using the trouble-shooting table opposite, you can analyse irregularities indicated by the engine instruments and perhaps remedy them with the means on board.

Instrument reading	Malfunction	Cause
Engine fails to reach design revs	Engine receiving insufficient air	Air filter dirty
		Leak in air-charging line
		Charge air cooling defective
	Fuel system defective	No fuel
		Water in fuel
		Air in fuel
		Fuel filter dirty
		Leak in fuel system
		Pump feeds too little/no fuel
		Overflow valve defective
		Injection pump/nozzles not working properly
Exhaust temp. deviates from normal value	Some cylinders cutting out	Broken valve spring(s)
		Inlet/exhaust valve sticking
		Valve clearance incorrect
		Injection nozzle defective
		Injection timing correct
Engine cooling water temp. too high		Cooling water pressurised
		Too little water in system
		Inadequate re-cooling
		Air in cooling water circuit
		Cooling circuit very dirty
		Thermostat defective
		Cooling fan control defective
		Cooling fan drive defective
		Thermometer defective
Engine oil temp. too high		Oil system heat exchanger dirty
	Oil pressure too low	Leak in system
		Oil filter dirty
		Pressure control valve defective
		Oil pump/drive damaged
		Fuel in the oil
		Too little oil in the sump
Oil pressure rises	Water in the oil	Oil heat exchanger leaks
		Cylinder liner leaks
		Cylinderhead leaks
		Crankcase leaks

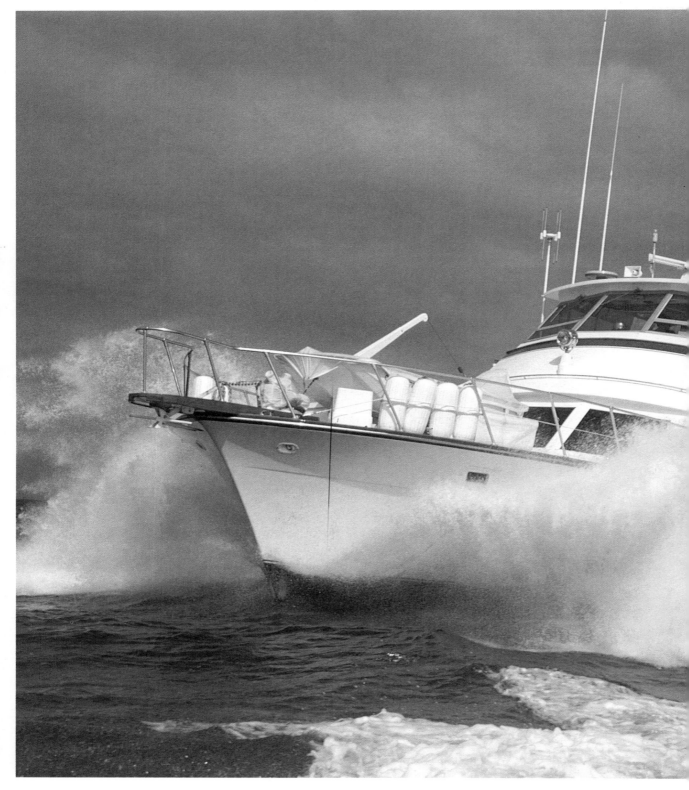

Motor boats – driving and manoeuvring

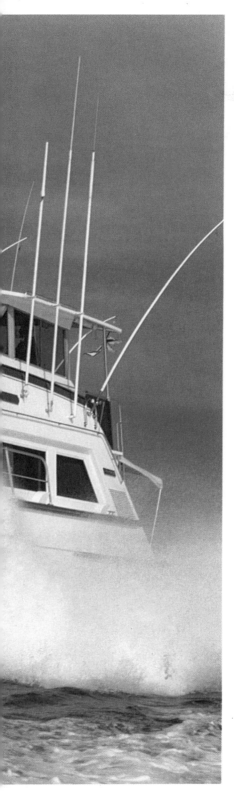

Newcomers to the water often believe that handling a motor boat is rather like driving a car. This impression tends to be strengthened by the fact that modern motor boat helm positions feel, to the uninitiated, a bit like car driving seats. In reality, though, driving and boat handling are worlds apart. The first difference which soon becomes apparent is that you cannot just jump into a boat and set off straightaway. There are various checks and preparations to be carried out before you are ready to cast off. Your engine is a much more vital piece of equipment afloat than it is on dry land and so, for your own safety, it needs careful looking after.

The first check when you get aboard is to make sure the bilges are dry and there are no signs of any oil leaks from the engine. The cooling water seacocks for inboard engines should have been turned off before you came ashore last time, so these need to be opened again. The fuel cock will have been turned off if the boat has a petrol engine, and maybe even if it has a diesel, so this needs to be turned on again. Make sure you look at the fuel level in the tank, either by using a dipstick or by checking the sight-tube or fuel gauge if fitted.

Check the engine oil dipstick and the gearbox oil. If the level of either has changed significantly since the last time you were on board, you must find out the cause before getting under way. Then a quick glance at the water separator. Water shows up as a greyish white sludge or as a separating line in the sight glass. Turn on the batteries at the master switch and make sure all the electrics are working.

On boats with outboard motors, make sure that the fuel tank is firmly secured to stop it shifting if conditions get choppy. Check the level in the tank and make sure that the engine isn't going to cough and die because, in the hurry to get away, you didn't open the vent screw in the top of the tank. Remember to squeeze the primer pump a few times before trying to start the engine, especially if the tank has just been connected. Finally check the engine clamping screws on the transom for tightness.

With inboard engines, run the engine compartment blower for at least 40 seconds to vent off any fumes which may have gathered since you last used the boat. And if your boat has an outdrive, don't forget to lower this into the water if, as is recommended, you normally leave it in the 'up' position.

Some starter systems have a safety interlock, so that you can only start up in neutral. Otherwise, make sure that the engine is out of gear before you turn the key. You should normally use the choke when cold starting a petrol engine. The equivalent for indirect

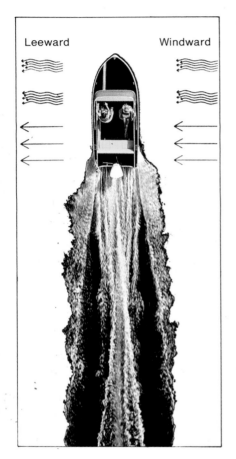

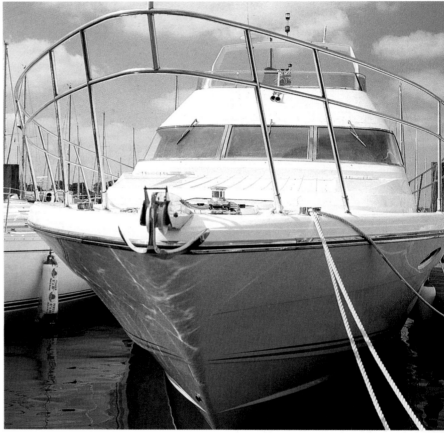

Windward side and leeward side except in a dead calm or still water, as soon as your boat starts moving you become involved with the effects of wind and current. By a tradition of the sea, the direction from which the wind is coming is called 'windward'; that in which it is going, 'leeward'. 'Upwind' and 'Downwind' are also used, and similarly 'upstream' and 'downstream'. The windward and leeward sides of a boat are the sides towards and away from the wind. Trouble can arise, for example when anchoring, from a lee shore to leeward of the yacht in an onshore wind. If the anchor doesn't hold, the boat will soon run aground.

In the diagram, **Leeward** is labelled at the top left and **Windward** at the top right.

injected diesels are the heater plugs operated by an intermediate position of the starter key. Direct injected diesels sometimes use heater plugs too, or there may be a cold start lever which results in extra diesel being injected until the engine is running.

Once the engine has started, it's worth letting it run at a fast idle in neutral for a few minutes to warm up. Don't overdo this though. Most engines are better off working under load as soon as they are warm enough to avoid the risk of stalling as you try to leave your berth.

Leaving a berth

Leaving a berth with an outboard engine or outdrive is perhaps more like driving a car than when manoeuvring with inboard engines. This is because an outboard or outdrive steers the boat very directly, by aiming the propeller thrust in the direction determined by the wheel. With inboard engined boats, on the other hand, the steering effect comes from the rudder which depends, in turn, on the boat's motion through the water.

It is usually easier to leave a quay-side or jetty stern-first, as shown in the diagrams opposite. This is because it's the stern which swings most when you are swinging a boat, with the axis of rotation about a third of the boat's length from the bow. So a boat cannot be driven away ahead from a quayside like a car pulling away from a pave-ment edge, because you can use only a very gradual amount of rudder with-out the stern swinging in and hitting the quay.

Wind and tide complicate matters further. As a rule, whether you are travelling ahead or astern, you main-tain better control of the boat by man-oeuvring against a tidal stream or river current. A fresh breeze is often trickier to deal with than a strong tide. The taller her superstructure and the shallower her draught, the more vul-nerable a motor yacht is to the effect of wind.

With most boats, it's the bows which tend to fall away first in any kind of cross-wind. The underwater profile of the hull is generally much shallower forward than aft and so this end of the boat offers less resistance of the sideways force of the wind. In pos-ition 2 opposite, for example, you'd have to be careful not to let your bow swing too close to the moored motor cruiser which is now close on your starboard side.

When manoeuvring outboard and outdrive boats, which have very posi-tive steering with the engine in gear but almost none with the engine in neutral, you have to co-ordinate the helm, gear-shift and throttle skilfully. If the wheel is hard over when you give a sudden burst of power, the stern will swing bodily to one side, perhaps rather faster than you'd expected. On

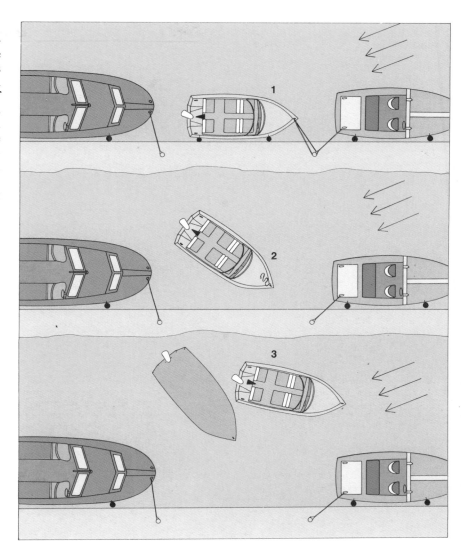

Leaving the jetty – wind on the bow (with outboard or outdrive)
1 Cast off stern warp, rig the bow warp as a slip, leave fenders out. Angle the drive towards the open water. Engage astern gear. Cast off bow warp.
2 The boat moves astern away from the jetty until it roughly reaches position.
3 Stop the engine. Leave the drive angled, go ahead and get on to your course.

With an offshore wind the manoeuvre is even easier. Push off the bow or the stern – depending on whether the wind is coming more from ahead or from astern – with your boathook or your feet. Using your hands to push off can be dangerous because that brings the body's centre of gravity outboard. When the bow/stern is some 15° to 20° out from the jetty, put the drive midships and go slow ahead/astern to get the boat clear of the jetty.

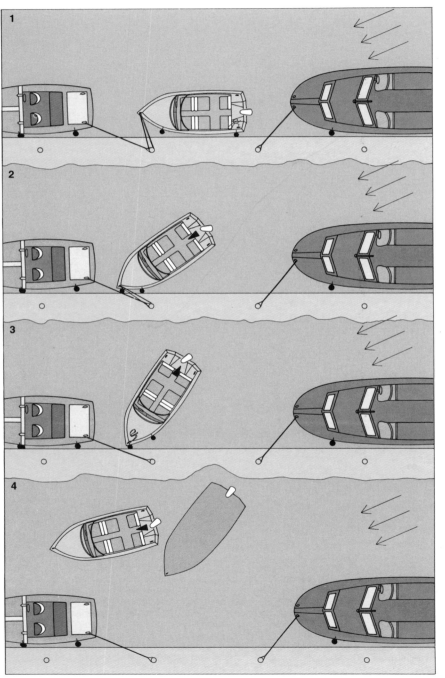

Leaving the jetty – wind on the quarter
(with outboard or outdrive)

1   Cast off stern warp, rig the bow warp as a slip to act as a spring. Put fenders out forward.

2   Angle the drive towards the jetty and motor ahead slowly. Possibly veer the spring a bit to provide enough play for the bow to pull around along the jetty.

3   When the stern of the boat is pointing roughly upwind, stop the engine and put the drive amidships. Cast off the spring and go astern to clear the jetty.

4   What happens now depends on the room for manoeuvre and the position of the jetty relative to the open water. Either go astern some more, or turn to port or starboard going ahead to get on to your course.

(With a fixed shaft the procedure is exactly the same. Instead of angling the drive, you angle the rudder. In position 3, when going astern it may be necessary to counter the paddlewheel effect using the rudder.)

the other hand, you often need to be quite positive about the application of power, especially in conditions where either you take charge or the wind does.

Because the helmsman may need to use sudden bursts of power when manoeuvring, the crew must be careful when moving about a lightweight boat to handle the ropes and fenders. Wherever possible, slipped mooring lines should be controlled from the cockpit of a small runabout, rather than from a slippery foredeck. Once the boat is safely clear of her berth and under way, the crew should then bring all fenders and ropes inboard and stow them carefully. Things are easier aboard larger boats where you can move safely around the deck, although the helmsman will want warps and fenders stowed quickly and the crew off the foredeck so that his view ahead is not obstructed.

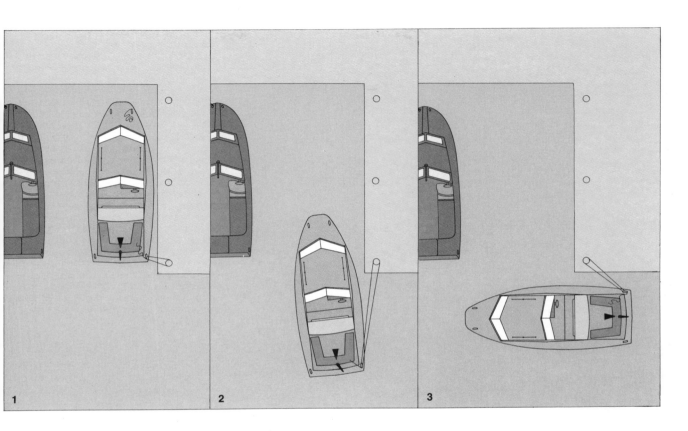

1

2

3

Fixed-shaft boats react less positively than outboards or outdrives, but can make effective use of the paddlewheel effect for their manoeuvres. They have a marked 'favoured side' for coming alongside and turning – the port side and clockwise turns with right-handed propellers, because the stern tends to swing to port when you put the engine in reverse to slow down. Of course this can result in certain difficulties when leaving berth, because now the non-favoured side is towards the open water. You will probably then need to use a spring to help escape from a quay, as shown in the diagram on page 72. If in doubt, the judicious use of a spring is more seamanlike than

vigorous backing and filling with frantic gear shifts and bursts of throttle. The latter is more likely to result in damage to your own boat and to others berthed nearby. However, to be able to go ahead on the spring the bow has to be well fendered, and sometimes the wide flare forward makes it necessary to use very large balloon fenders. Turning just on the rubbing strake is rarely practical because few rubbing strakes are strong enough to take the forces involved.

Life is much easier for twin-engined yachts. With their contra-rotating props and ability to pivot almost in their own length, it doesn't usually matter whether they berth port side-to or starboard side-to.

Turning on the spring
If you have to leave a tight berth backwards and then turn in the direction which is awkward for a fixed-shaft boat (here, a right-handed prop), there is only one way to do it:
1 Cast off the bow warp, rig the stern warp as a slip to act as a spring. Rudder midships, slow astern. Veer the spring as necessary.
2 Stop the spring. Angle the rudder towards the jetty and bring the boat into position.
3 Recover the spring smartly, rudder midships and go ahead.
The spring should, if possible, be manned from the jetty by a crew-member who is picked up again in position 3.

73

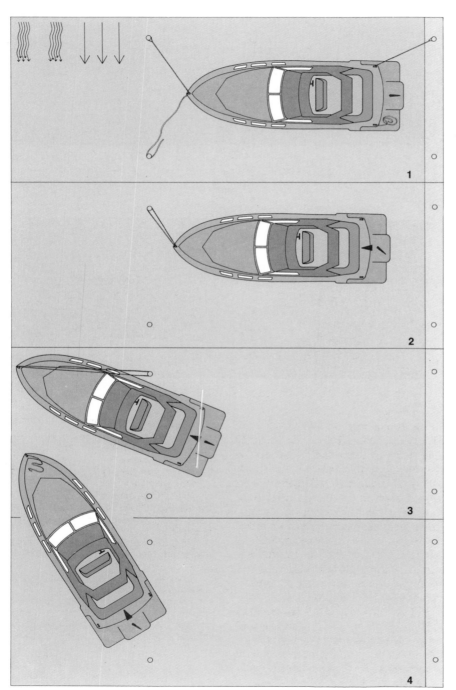

Leaving a pile berth – wind or current on the beam
1   Start the engine, cast off the leeward stern line. Veer both windward lines and haul the boat, or let it drift, over to the leeward pile. Cast off the leeward bow line. Haul the boat back to windward using the two windward lines and rig the bow line as a slip.
2   Cast off the stern line and haul it in quickly to prevent it fouling the prop. Angle the drive slightly to leeward to counter the wind or current pressure on the stern. Slow ahead. Keep the bow line taut, veering it only as necessary for the forward travel of the boat. Watch out; don't let the bow sheer off to leeward.
3   The bow line has been veered to about $\frac{2}{3}$ of the length of the boat, the stern is clear of the leeward pile. Stop the engine.
4   Angle the drive towards the pivot pile and go slow ahead. Cast off bow line and recover quickly to prevent it fouling the prop. At cruising speed, turn on to your course.

Out of the pile berth with twin engines (wind on the quarter)
1   Cast off the leeward stern line, rudder to windward. Cast off windward stern line. Windward engine ahead. Leeward engine about half-speed astern, as a counter.
2   Leeward engine ahead; throttle back windward. Veer leeward bow line as necessary. Haul taut windward bow line and bring the stern to the leeward pile. Cast off leeward bow line.
3   Cast off windward bow line; leeward rudder. Both engines ahead and swiftly bring the boat out from between the piles.

If in position 2 you get turned strongly sideways, run the windward engine faster to increase the effect of the rudder. Skilful throttle jugglers carry out manoeuvres like this purely on the engines; the rudder remains untouched amidships.

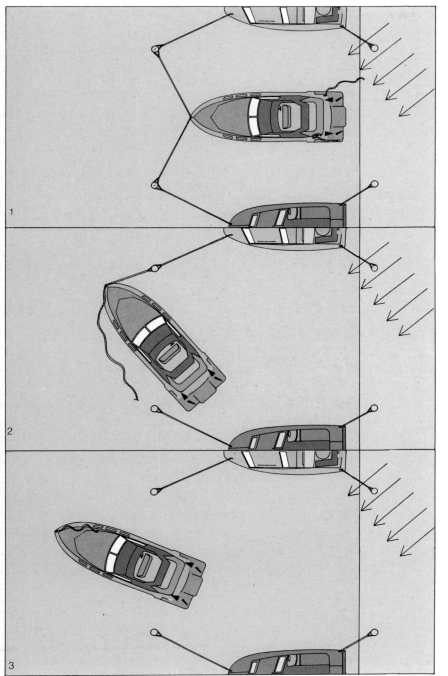

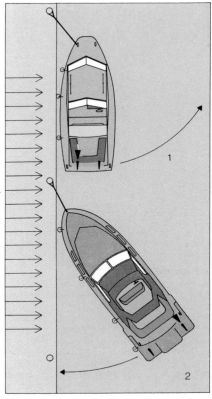

Leaving and coming alongside with twin engines

1 Leaving a jetty or pier, you run the inside engine astern. The rudder remains amidships. The strong turning effect of the off-centre prop makes the stern swing out into the fairway. With an outdrive you use the same technique.

2 Coming alongside, you leave the outside engine running astern, the rudder amidships. The turning effect pulls the stern in. Only in a strong offshore wind (as here) do you have to hang from a bow line.

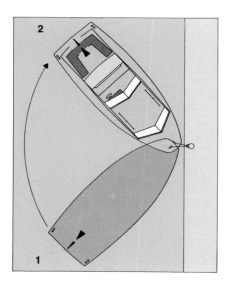

Powering against warps
(with a right-handed prop)
Cast off all lines except the hitched-short bow warp. With the rudder amidships and engine going astern, the paddle-wheel effect will pull the boat round 180°. Swinging the stern round like this can also make sense if you are lying between two posts or mooring buoys and want to leave with the wind or the current on the quarter.

Leaving a buoy

This really ought not to present any problems at all. You rig the bow warp as a slip and, with the engine out of gear, let the boat drop astern until you are sure of being clear of the buoy tackle. Only then do you cast off the bow warp, engage the propeller and go ahead on course.

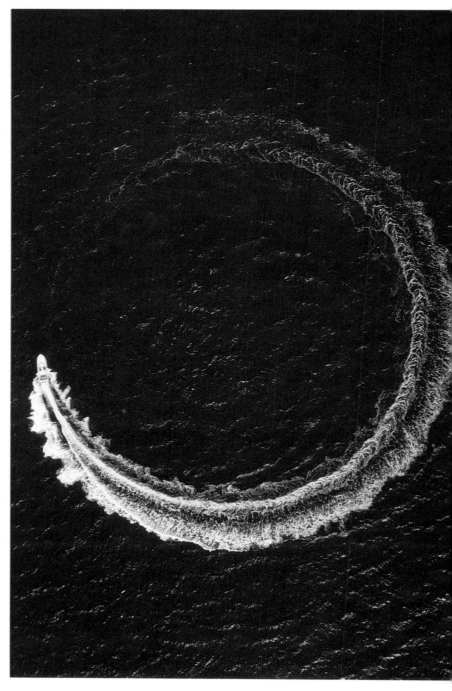

Going ahead, astern and into a turn

Driving a motor boat is a bit of a mystery. Every boat behaves differently – and some don't behave at all, at least that's how it sometimes seems to beginners. But once you have practised a few of the basics and begun to appreciate how propeller and rudder work together, manoeuvring becomes great fun and highly satisfying. Of course everyone has to gain a certain amount of experience with a new or strange boat in order to master it properly. Motor boats don't have any brakes to take way off and bring them to rest – to do this you shift into reverse. When you do this, boats with a single fixed propeller swing to one side because of the paddlewheel effect. For that reason, but also for the sake of the transmission, it is important to avoid the need for decelerating fiercely.

The angle swept by the rudder blade is normally limited to between 35° and 55° on either side. Avoiding oversteer in a given situation is a matter of the driver's 'feel' for the boat. If you put the rudder over too far at the wrong moment while manoeuvring, the boat will react badly. It's particularly easy to get this wrong going astern, with the result that the steering effect disappears altogether. An expert helmsman uses the helm as little as possible when turning, increasing the rudder angle progressively until full rudder is finally reached. Too little rudder makes the turn painfully slow; too much, on the other hand, can make a botch of a planned manoeuvre.

Different types of boats behave in different ways when you steer to make a turn. Different hull shapes and

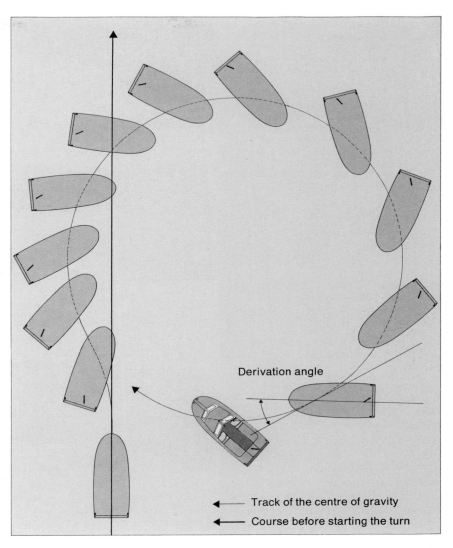

Derivation angle

Track of the centre of gravity

Course before starting the turn

This is roughly how the minimum turning circle turn of a single engined fixed-shaft boat looks from beginning to end. The angular difference during this manoeuvre between the boat's centreline and a tangent to the turning circle is known as the derivation angle.

A sharp turn with a planing craft and out-drive, at about $\frac{3}{4}$ power – it always looks more spectacular from outside than it actually is. The derivation angle is much smaller than that of a fixed-shaft boat, the turning circle tighter. Because the pivot-point is far aft, the boat banks impressively; the underwater hull assumes an angle of attack – an inclined plane – relative to the water. The more pronounced the 'V', the more one slides 'on the cheek'. Boats with poor hull design sometimes tend to 'dig in' and can't easily be brought back on to a straight course by means of the rudder.

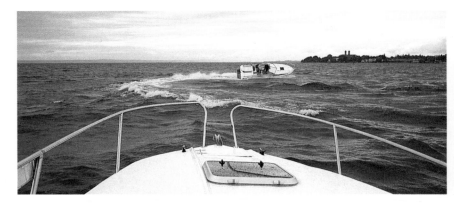

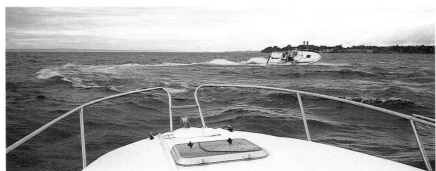

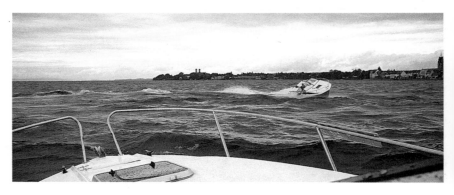

underwater profiles lead to markedly different locations for the axis of rotation. Displacement craft normally turn about the forward third of the boat, fixed-shaft planing craft have their axis of rotation about amidships, and outboard or outdrive planing craft have it roughly in the after third. In the case of displacement craft the stern swings in a much larger arc than the bow, and the boat often heels outwards – at high speed even ominously. A planing craft behaves somewhat like a sleigh in the bends of a bobsleigh run: it heels inwards and builds up a 'banking' of water, slipping sideways to the outer edge of the bend to produce a flat elliptical curve. If you turn sharply in a planing craft to avoid an obstacle, you could unexpectedly land

on top of it if you don't allow for the sideways slide. There are boats which, in a fast sharp turn, tend to 'lock in' ie you can't pull them out of the turn easily and back on to a straight course. This is sometimes a critical situation which can end in a capsize. Nothing for it but to throttle right back, at once. The same applies if the prop starts to ingest air. The engine screams and the boat all of a sudden loses way. But most boats can cope with turns even at full throttle, as long as they are not seriously over-powered

to start with. Mind you, a beginner shouldn't start with high-speed turns, but rather should get the feel of the turning circle by increasing the revs gradually. That's the best way of establishing a relationship with, and confidence in, your boat. Although you shouldn't make a habit of high-speed sharp turns however, the need may arise if you suddenly have to avoid a swimmer or some debris in the water. You should always take great care when using your boat near holiday beaches.

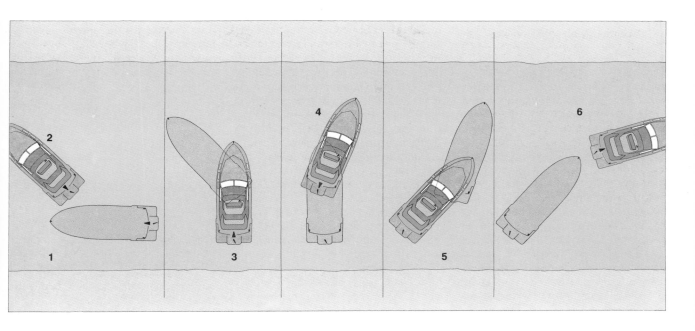

Turning in a restricted space

With a single-screw boat, this is possibly the most important of all manoeuvres to master. To be able to turn in a restricted space requires a careful understanding of the combined effects of propeller and rudder. Time and again you will need to turn your boat in crowded yacht harbours, in order to get safely into a pontoon berth or perhaps to escape from a line of pontoons while you are looking for an empty berth. Always start the turn in the direction of rotation of the propeller, ie to starboard if your propeller is right-handed because the stern will swing naturally to port when going astern and assist the turn. The paddlewheel effect when driving astern makes it possible to turn in a narrower space than the boat's normal turning circle when driving ahead. Two points are important:

1 The boat's immediate reaction to a short, sharp burst ahead when carrying helm is to turn but gather very little way. Of course you mustn't wait until the boat does gather way before shifting astern, otherwise the turning circle will get correspondingly larger. And after shifting gear don't be too timid with the throttle, particularly not when going astern.

2 A short, sharp burst astern produces a strong sideways movement of the stern because of the paddlewheel effect, and the rudder then has relatively little effect by comparison. The boat comes to a stop and then gathers sternway only slowly.

Turning in a narrow space
1 With a right-handed prop start near the port side of your turning area, going slowly. Starboard rudder. The boat turns into position.
2 Half astern until the way is off the boat and it starts to go astern. The rudder stays to starboard – it has no steering effect now. The paddlewheel effect of the backwards-running prop turns the boat roughly into position.
3 Stop. Half ahead to take off the sternway, until the boat roughly reaches position.
4 Half astern. The rudder still stays to starboard. The paddlewheel effect of the backwards-running prop pushes the stern roughly into position.
5 Stop. Half ahead. Rudder midships and come on to course (6).

Turning twin-engined yachts

Turning in a restricted space with twin engines is much more straightforward. You go ahead with the 'outer' prop and astern with the 'inner'. The boat's turn matches the control lever movement, so if you've pushed the starboard lever forwards and the port lever astern, then in a manner of speaking, the starboard side of the yacht moves ahead and the port side comes astern; ie the boat turns to the left. By careful use of differing revs for each engine, the boat can be turned literally in its own length. Because a propeller is less efficient when going astern, the engine in reverse must be run a little faster than the engine driving ahead. The rudder remains amidships. Contrary to a widespread belief, the distance of the prop shafts from the centreline does not appreciably affect the boat's manoeuvring qualities. What is more important is the underwater profile of the hull and the way in which the boat's bottom divides into port and starboard zones either side of the keel along the deadrise.

Should your rudders become defective during a trip, you can drive twin-engined yachts home by steering with the throttles. The trick is to set the desired revs on the windward engine and then steer with the leeward throttle, opening or closing it as necessary. You can hold a pretty steady course that way. Nevertheless you should make for the nearest harbour, because all that fiddling with the throttle mops up the fuel and reduces your range considerably.

Turns with two props: going ahead with one engine (1 – 2) produces a gentler turn than going astern with the other (3 – 4) in the same direction. Useful to remember and allow for when manoeuvring in tight corners.

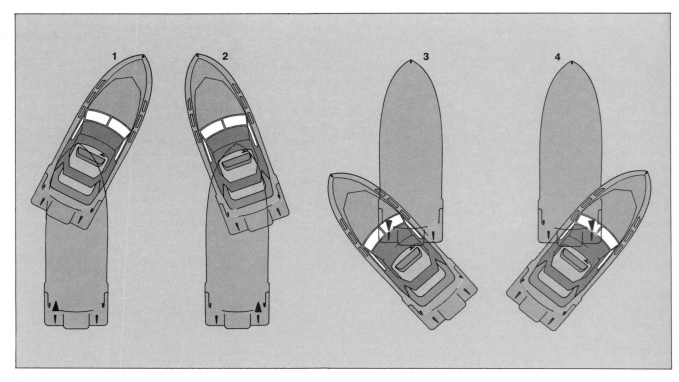

The emergency stop

Situations can, of course, arise where you have to stop unexpectedly from full speed. With a single-screw boat, you will probably end up at an angle of about 90° to your original direction of travel, whatever you do with the helm. The explanation is simple – the more power you apply when going astern to stop quickly, the more powerful the paddlewheel effect. For as long as you have enough forward way on, the boat obeys the rudder normally. As the way is lost, the rudder becomes less effective and finally goes dead whereas the swing applied to the stern by the paddle-wheel effect continues all the more strongly. For turning in a restricted space this behaviour, with the braking effect of going astern, the paddlewheel effect and the boat's angular momentum all working together, can be very useful. But for an emergency stop it can mean the boat going temporarily out of control. Heavy displacement craft, when crash-stopping like this, may swing up to 180° about their axis. The remedy is simple. As with driving on the road, always travel at a safe speed so that you can slow down and stop gradually under full control.

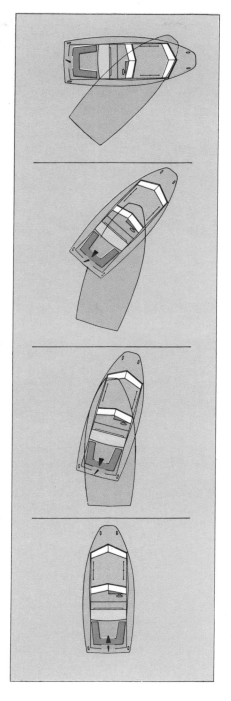

How the boat lies after an emergency stop – slewed across the direction of advance by momentum and paddle-wheel effect.

Going astern

Outdrive boats running slowly sometimes have trouble holding a straight line when going astern. Generally speaking, however, they pull the boat fairly accurately in the direction in which they are pointed. Fixed shaft single prop boats never behave like that; they invariably try to turn away to one side. That can't be helped. During lengthy runs astern, it may be necessary to straighten the boat up by making short bursts ahead with the rudder well over, so that the boat gathers no headway, or only very little, but then comes back on line. Then carry on going astern slowly until the same game starts again.

You have to be careful about applying rudder when going astern quickly because the rudder tends to be forced 'hard over' and is then subject to great strain. A novice helmsman may even have the wheel torn out of his hands. So you should make it a basic rule to go astern only slowly, at about one quarter throttle.

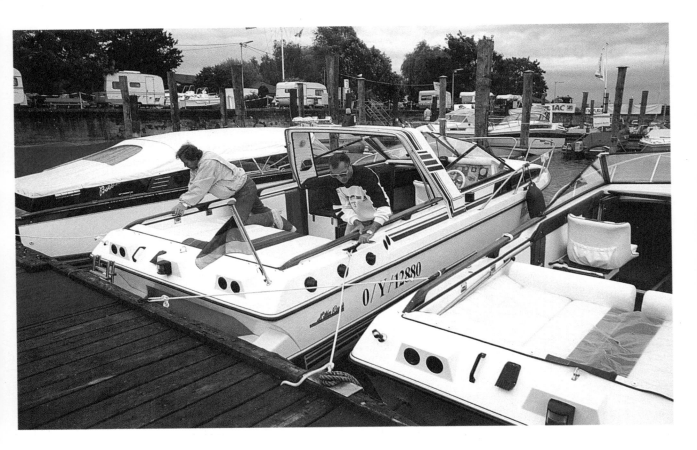

Going alongside

Competent boat handlers are made, not born. Of course there are people with something like an inborn feel for how vessels behave – they will always make betters helmsmen – but, in the main, skill is based on experience. In other words, practice makes perfect. After not driving a boat for the whole of a winter though, it's quite easy to get a bit rusty. Lucky the boat owner who can find a quiet deserted stretch of water where he can have a couple of unobserved practice runs at creeping slowly up to a jetty, check the effect of

going astern and going ahead, experiment with the stopping distance and the swing of the stern, decide whether or not to apply power, and so on. Such care is particularly needed if you have recently changed from a boat with a steered prop to a fixed shaft, or from a twin prop to a single prop craft.

For going alongside, you should use only as much power as you need to remain manoeuvrable. At some distance from the jetty you should go into neutral, because at idling revs with the engine in gear many boats still move much faster than one would think. Always remember that it is easier to speed up than to slow down.

One of the great skills of boat handling is the art of 'hovering' while you are working out where to berth, or perhaps waiting for a boat already alongside a quay to pull away. You slip out of gear for a while and let the boat lose way, keeping some helm on to counteract the effect of any wind or tide. Then, before the boat becomes difficult to control, you nudge into gear again to maintain steerage way.

As a rule, if at all possible, you should approach a berth by heading into the wind or current. If these two elements are coming from opposite directions, head into that which affects the boat most strongly. In the

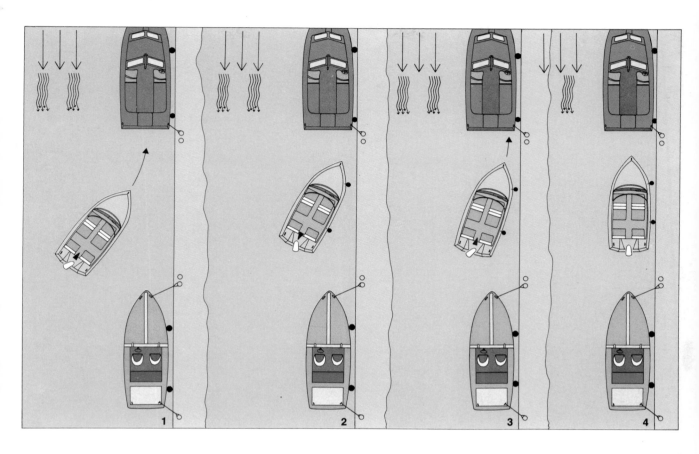

case of a motor yacht with a high superstructure, that will usually be the wind. Having the wind or current from ahead helps to stop the boat naturally, whereas a wind or current from astern when berthing adds unwanted thrust which can only complicate matters.

During berthing, crew in small lightweight craft must absolutely stay put, because shifts of weight, whether lengthways or athwartships, can alter the behaviour of the boat unpredictably and may well spoil the berthing manoeuvre that the driver has carefully worked out.

Once you have eased alongside and

Coming alongside against current and wind

1 At as acute an angle as possible, run to within half a boat's length (barely) of the berth. Go into neutral.
2 Angle the drive towards the jetty and engage astern gear. The boat is first stopped, then starts to drop astern, the stern moving towards the jetty.
3 Stop the engine. Angle the drive the other way. Go ahead. The stern swings towards the jetty, the boat starts to make headway.
4 Drive midships, stop the engine. If current or wind don't stop the boat at once, give a short burst astern with the engine.

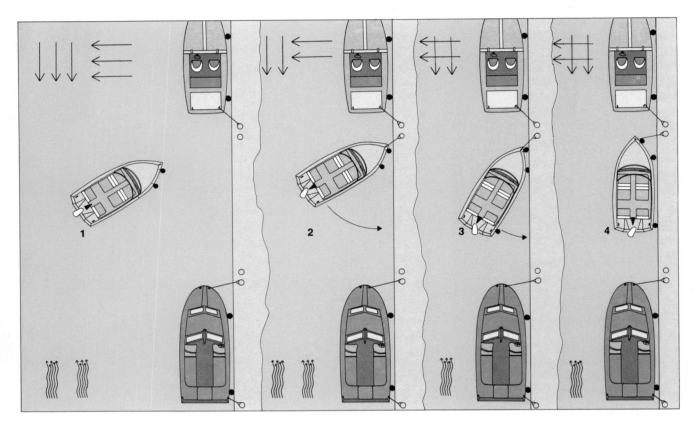

Coming alongside with wind or current complicating matters

Either wind and current are opposed parallel to the jetty, or there is a strong wind from the jetty.

1 Head for the jetty at a broad angle. Rig hefty fenders forward. Stop the engine or give a short burst astern.

2 Get the bow warp ashore. Angle the drive towards the jetty. Go slowly astern.

3 The stern is pulled towards the jetty, the bow prevented from sheering off by the bow warp. Veer this only enough to allow the bow to turn.

4 When the boat is roughly parallel to the jetty, opposite rudder briefly to arrest the turn. Stop the engine. Make fast the stern warp.

given the engine a touch astern to bring the boat to a stop, get the bow line ashore first if the wind or current is coming from ahead, or the stern line if wind or current is coming from astern. Although one usually tries to avoid coming alongside *with* the wind or current, this sometimes can't be avoided. When you are entering a lock, for example, the wind may be funnelling in behind you, or a quiet but steady current might be running through the lock and over the far gates. In this case you will have to get the stern line ashore quickly or the stern will start to swing out at once, and there'll be little hope of avoiding a collision with any boat lying ahead.

Whether berthing or leaving a berth, lines should never be hand-held directly but always held via a turn around a cleat or a bollard. Friction then provides a major part of the holding force. Well before berthing the skipper should explain his intended manoeuvre carefully to the crew so that everyone knows what they are supposed to do. Any crew member not participating in the manoeuvre should sit well back out of the driver's view, or perhaps go below in a larger boat.

Mooring in marina berths is often done stern-first, which then makes it easier to get ashore. However, anyone still a little unsure about their berthing technique can always enter the berth bow-first to make things easier. When planning to leave again there'll be more time to work out how best to carry out the manoeuvre, and perhaps not quite so many spectators.

Things are different if you have to anchor and make fast stern-to a jetty, as is frequently the case in the Mediterranean. Be warned – do not moor with an anchor out astern and your bow towards the pier. Should an onshore wind suddenly blow up – and that happens quite frequently – you are then in a vulnerable position with your exposed stern towards the weather.

The anchor doesn't always hold in such circumstances, particularly since all too often it gets tangled with others. Is there anyone who has not had the experience of raising two other anchors as well as your own when wanting to get under way?

Bollards in the Mediterranean may be of reinforced concrete, which will soon chafe through even the best of lines. So for anything more than a short stay, arm the ends of your stern warps with a length of stout chain. Crossed stern warps help stop the stern swinging which is useful if boats are packed fairly close together. In tidal harbours where the water level varies significantly, the stern warps must not be too short or the after end of the boat will hang from them. You are strongly recommended to use a buoyed tripping line fastened to the crown of your anchor. This not only helps you recover the anchor again when the time comes, but it also discourages others from putting theirs down in the same place.

Things are less complicated in the more modern yacht harbours and marinas of the Mediterranean, where

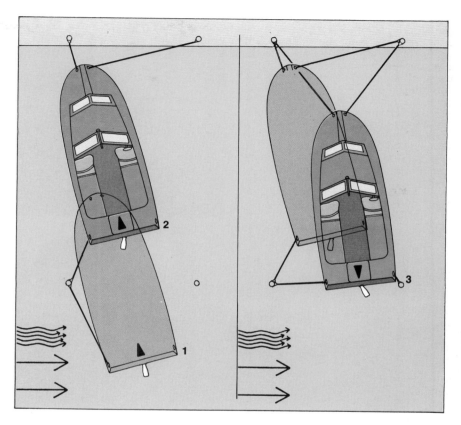

fixed moorings are used instead of your own anchor. The cables are lying on the bottom and need only be fished up with a boathook and belayed. This is a practical arrangement, although the mooring will often be slimey when it comes on board. When making lines fast ashore, don't leave any more rope on the quayside bollard or cleat than is needed for belaying. Any surplus rope should always be taken aboard and coiled. Although it is convenient to leave any permanent, cut-to-length bow or stern wraps on top of the bollard when leaving the berth, the next strong gust of wind may blow them into the water where they then lurk, waiting to trap your propeller.

Entering the pile berth with a side wind or current
1 Approach the windward pile at an acute angle, angle the drive slightly to windward and rig a spring from the stern. Go ahead. Haul the spring taut as necessary to stop the stern sheering off.
2 Use windward rudder to balance the lateral current/wind pressure on the stern. Stop the engine. First make fast the windward bow line, then run out the leeward one. Rig both bow lines as slips so that they can be veered from on board.
3 Drive angled towards the leeward pile, go astern on the engine to pull the stern towards this. Stop the engine. Rig the leeward stern line. Adjust the lines by hand to position the boat correctly in the berth. Switch off the engine.

Entering a pile berth with an outdrive
(the wind coming from the side)

Slowly run past the berth until you are about halfway past the leeward pile (1). Take off the way. Rudder towards the leeward pile, a sharp burst astern (2) and turn around the pile – perhaps rubbing against it. Simultaneously rig the bow line – better still, both bow lines (3). Continue turning into the berth. If necessary, straighten the boat with a short burst ahead – that's just been done here as you can see from the wake (4) – and drop astern until you reach the jetty. With an outdrive (or outboard) it's rare to need lines to help you with manoeuvres like this.

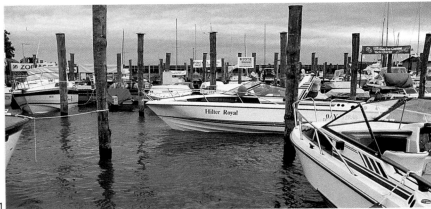

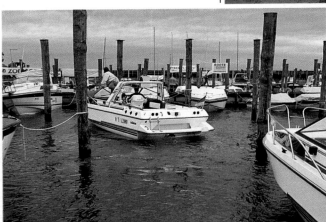

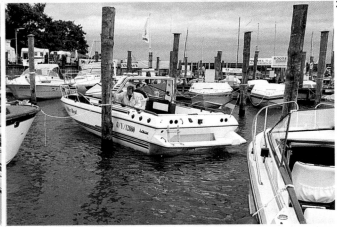

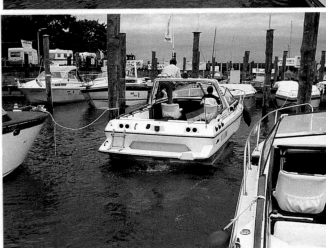

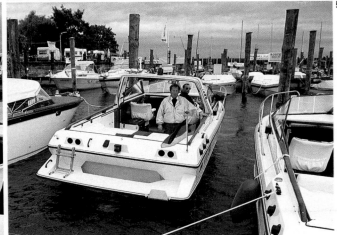

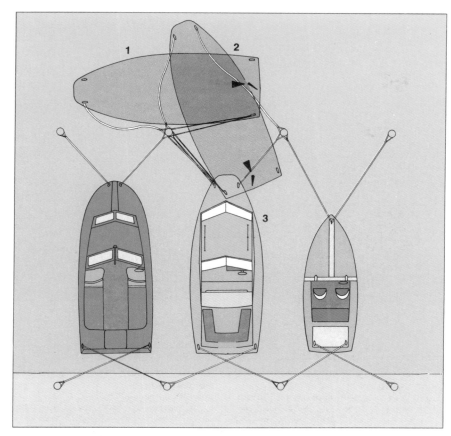

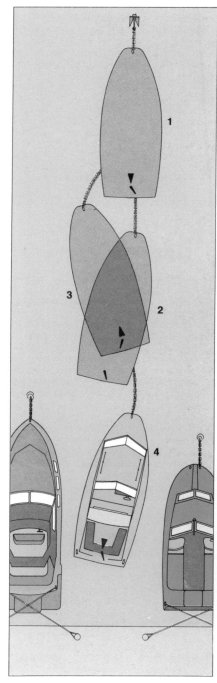

Turning into a pile berth
(whatever the wind direction)

1   Approach the pile at an acute angle, going slowly. Stop the engine or give a short burst astern and first take a stern spring to the pile, then the port (in this case) bow line.

2   Slow astern, rudder towards the pile and stop the spring at about half the boat's length. The boat turns on the spring. Veer the bow line as necessary, take the starboard bow line to its pile.

3   Let go the spring – or if the wind is from the port side leave it – and drop astern to the jetty controlled by the bow lines. Stop the engine, make fast the stern warps. Crossed stern warps prevent the stern swinging in cross-winds.

A safe manoeuvre in a restricted space. If your rubbing strake is stout enough, lay the boat alongside the pile; the rubbing contact speeds up the turn.

Anchoring stern-to a wall

1   At a distance, depending on the depth of water in the harbour which makes safe anchoring possible, drop the bow anchor in line with the free berth. Motor astern. To balance the paddlewheel effect of a right-handed prop, apply slight starboard rudder.

2   The stern runs out to port.

3   Engine in neutral, port rudder. With a short burst ahead, swing the bow across the course line. Stop the engine as soon as the boat starts to go ahead. Starboard rudder, go astern. Halfway into the berth, snub the cable and give more astern power to make sure the anchor bites.

4   Paying out the cable some more, let the engine pull you astern to the pier. If the stern starts to swing to port again, give another burst ahead to correct the paddlewheel effect.

As we have seen here, it is usually difficult with a single-prop, fixed-shaft boat to go astern over any distance in a roughly straight line.

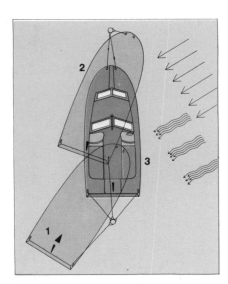

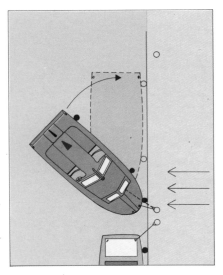

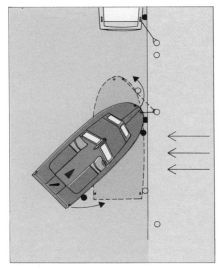

Mooring between two piles or mooring buoys

(wind/current from starboard side; prop right-handed)

1 Approach the downstream pile upwind and make fast the stern warp.

2 Pay out stern warp, run on to the upstream pile, correct the heading using the rudder and make fast the bow warp.

3 Haul/pay out the warps until the boat is the same distance from both piles (or buoys).

With wind (current) from the port side, make the initial approach to the upstream pile, make fast the bow warp and then motor astern to pull the boat to the downstream pile.

Coming alongside against an offshore wind or current

(boat with fixed shaft and normal rudder)

If possible, come alongside 'favoured side-to', ie port side-to with a right-handed prop.

1 Approach at an angle of about 45° with plenty of fenders out forward. Bow warp ashore. Rudder amidships – it has no effect – and astern on the engine.

2 The paddlewheel effect tucks the stern alongside the jetty.

Coming alongside against an offshore wind or current

(non-favoured side-to)

1 Approach at an angle of about 45°, plenty of fenders out forward, bow warp ashore. Rudder towards the open water, slow ahead.

2 The stern pulls the boat around, turning the bow warp into a bow spring.

Were you to motor astern in this situation, the paddlewheel effect would pull the stern away from the jetty. The rudder would still be ineffective.

Made fast alongside the jetty

If you're expecting to stay some time, rig a bow and a stern spring in addition to the bow and stern warps. They stop the boat from surging and prevent the bow or stern from sheering off, which would otherwise happen with a wind or current from forward or aft. Make fenders fast at the right height, so that they can't get pushed up on to the deck or the jetty (pier) and so become useless.

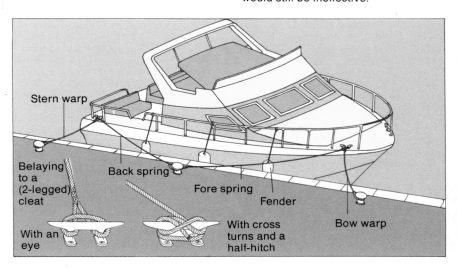

Stern warp

Belaying to a (2-legged) cleat

Back spring

Fore spring

Fender

Bow warp

With an eye

With cross turns and a half-hitch

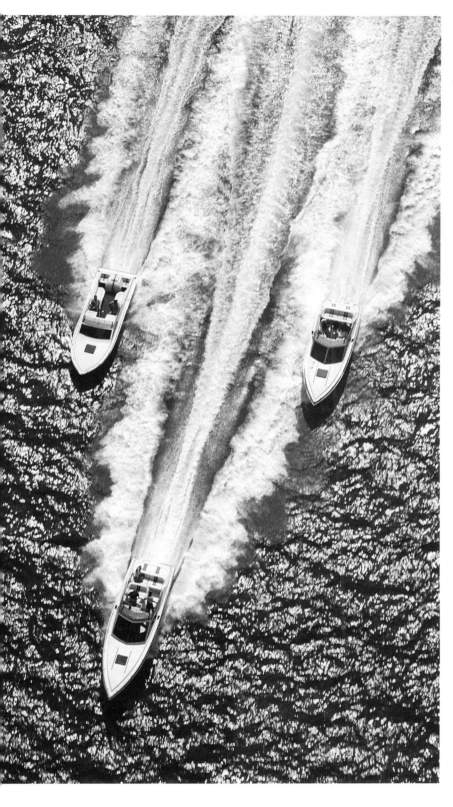

Adjusting your trim

Planing craft with a well matched hull and engine normally cruise with a glide-angle (the angle between the bottom of the boat and the water surface) of 2° to 4°. Semi-displacement craft have a glide angle of about 6°. Having the bow tilted up at more than this is inefficient and usually increases fuel consumption.

Now, it's a fact that smallish, lightweight planing craft are exceedingly sensitive to lengthways distribution of weight. Having all the passengers in an outboard boat sitting on the stern seats, or the bow tank in a day-cruiser either full or almost empty, can radically affect the trim. With poor trim, if the stern is tucked down for example, the revs drop, the boat goes more slowly, and fuel consumption increases. The simplest countermeasure is usually to transfer weight forward, perhaps by restowing anchor gear, any spare cans, or heavy holiday luggage. Also, the longitudinal trim can be influenced by the drive angle of the outboard or the outdrive leg.

It's more fun in company, particularly with boats trimmed so perfectly. Each hull touches the water about halfway along its length. The spray fans out sideways low down and the wash is minimal. That makes it possible for the other two boats to track the leading one precisely, cruising in its bow wave as you can see from the wake. From the shadow underneath the nose of each boat, you can see that the planing angle of the right-hand 'flank man' is a bit flatter. By the same token, the spray shoots out from a little further forward. The aerial photograph highlights such minor differences in trim.

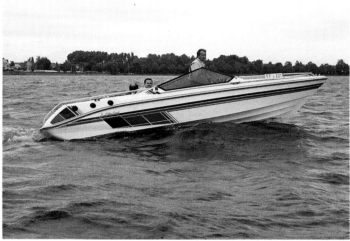

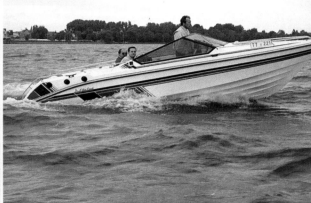

1

2

Above: **A heavy stern has trouble getting going**

1 The boat is running very slowly in displacement mode and is trimmed too low by the stern.

2 At about half revs, the stern is way down and the boat is being shoved along inefficiently. A sensible trim, however, for a small open boat in heavy seas, to stop the bow digging in.

3 A boat trimmed down by the stern as much as this has a job bringing the nose down again and getting on to the plane. Here a laborious planing mode has been achieved at about $\frac{3}{4}$ power. The afterbody is further out of the water – a sign of increasing dynamic buoyancy.

4 Now the boat is planing properly.

Right: **The correct angle of incidence for the outboard**

1 The engine is tilted too much. The bow is pushed upwards; a part of the prop's thrust is directed downwards. If the engine is heavy, behaviour under way may become erratic.

2 The optimum angle of incidence for planing. The prop can convert all its power into thrust ahead; the boat is cruising parallel to the surface and makes good speed and fuel economy.

3 The engine is pulled in too close to the transom. The bow is pushed down and is liable to dig in at sea.

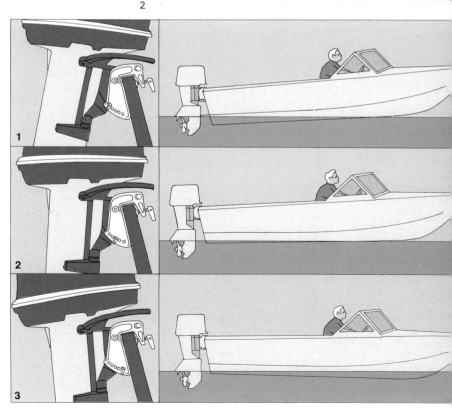

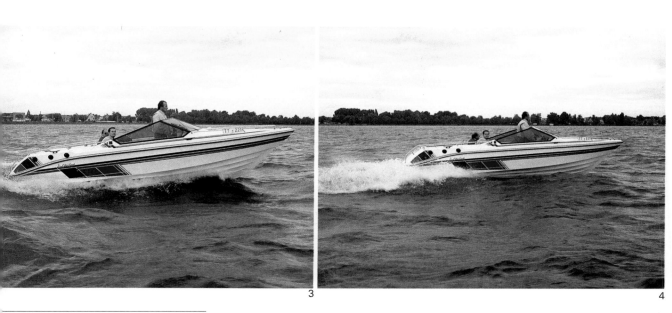

3

4

Trimming with an outboard or outdrive

The first mistakes which result in the boat not running correctly are sometimes made right at the start, when hanging the outboard from the transom. One leg of the outboard's tilting bracket is usually fitted with 4 or 5 trimming slots, which with the aid of a socket pin can be used to alter the drive angle of the shaft. When planing, the shaft should be perpendicular to the water surface – only then can the prop develop its thrust fully. Usually, the pin in the second hole from the front achieves that, the shaft being at an angle of 6° to 8° to the vertical with the boat at rest. Frequently a suggested setting is given in the engine operating manual, but of course this cannot be correct for all boats and their full range of loads.

Only trimming runs can establish the ideal setting for the engine shaft. At the same planing revs but with the pin in different holes, you carry out several runs over a measured distance and check the times. The shortest time indicates the ideal trim angle and the most economical operating conditions. The heavyweight, high powered outboards have hydraulic adjusting equipment, the 'powertrim' which, as with outdrive units, permits finger-tip control of the engine setting angle from the helming position.

If the engine is tilted too far away from the transom, the stern will be pushed down too far into the water. That increases the immersed surface, which in turn increases the frictional resistance and you may use as much as 12% more fuel. The effect of having the shaft *too close* to the transom is that the prop uses up part of its thrust to lift up the stern of the boat while the bow ploughs through the water. It therefore takes a lot longer, and correspondingly more fuel, to get planing. With less powerful engines, where you would normally only just get on the plane, you may not get there

at all. However, given sufficient power, these same effects can be used positively to improve longitudinal trim, where, for example, you need to lift an overloaded stern or the bow is pressed down into the water by an excess of gear loaded well forward. The effect of trim changes can be established by differential loading. In this case, you carry out a straight run at about 80% nominal revs and then ask one, or perhaps several, of the passengers to move forward or aft. If the trim change increases the revs, that means more speed and less fuel; if it reduces them, it means the opposite. Using 'live ballast' in this way allows you to check the effect on trim of correspondingly stowed baggage and gear for a lengthy trip, and establish the best engine setting for this. Should there be no significant rev changes either upwards or downwards, you are assured of starting out with an ideally trimmed boat.

Trim can, of course, be affected positively by changing the engine

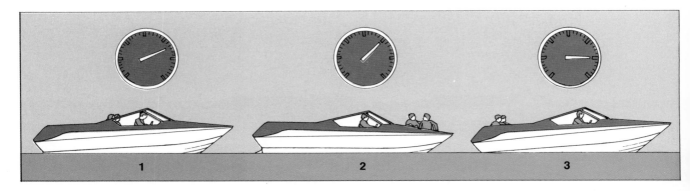

| 1 | 2 | 3 |

Use 'live ballast' to establish the best trim (for when you have to stow holiday luggage):
1 Three people all around the helming position – a balanced trim, you would think. But is it?

2 Two people (record the respective weights of the two trimmers) up forward. The revs drop, so was the first trim right after all?

3 Two people aft on the stern bench. That the rev counter needle has gone up further than it was at '1' indicates optimum trim. The boat in this example likes to be trimmed a bit down by the stern.

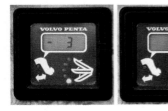

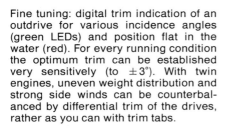

Fine tuning: digital trim indication of an outdrive for various incidence angles (green LEDs) and position flat in the water (red). For every running condition the optimum trim can be established very sensitively (to ±3°). With twin engines, uneven weight distribution and strong side winds can be counterbalanced by differential trim of the drives, rather as you can with trim tabs.

attitude only if the power available is not too little to get the boat planing properly, or the load so heavy that the propeller can no longer develop the necessary thrust. No amount of trimming will help them; only a more powerful engine or a prop with lower pitch.

Using trim tabs

Trim tabs lengthen the waterline and increase longitudinal stability. They are intended to give the stern more buoyancy and press down the bow, to make it easier for the boat to clamber over its own bow wave and achieve the ideal planing attitude as quickly as possible. Mind you, they can do that only in the so-called dynamic buoyancy zone, at speeds exceeding 25 km/h; at lower speeds they have no effect. Trim tabs, in the opinion of one

renowned motor boat builder, are no more than crutches for unsuccessful designs. You can certainly use trim tabs to improve matters if a badly designed hull won't run properly. But there are various reasons why some yards routinely fit trim tabs. For a start, if there is too little power for the size and weight of boat, trim tabs can help to overcome the nerve-racking hurdle before the hull gets on the plane. Sometimes there is too much engine weight aft, where heavy inboard engines have been installed in boats too small for them, particularly where the hull may well have been designed for a much lighter outboard engine. This may depress the stern so much that the trim can no longer be rectified by the engine setting angle. Similar problems may arise where 6-cylinder turbo-diesels are installed in boats intended only for lightweight petrol engines. In those cases too, the addition of trim tabs may be useful to

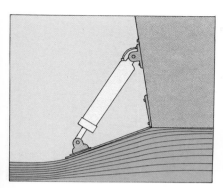

The trim tab along the transom operates similarly to an aircraft's elevator. Angled downwards, it lifts the stern of the boat and prevents it assuming progressively more of a 'hill-climbing' attitude as speed increases.

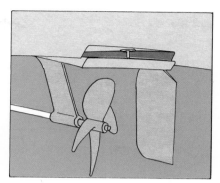

Adjustable chock: less delicate, but also less effective, than trim tabs.

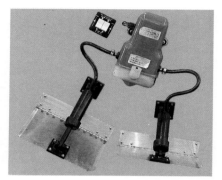

A trim tab assembly with motor and rocker switch mounted, for demonstration purposes, on the wall of a show stand. The left tab is fully depressed, the right one at zero setting. This combination of settings would counteract a strong heel to port.

achieve a better planing attitude.

However, trim tabs fitted to properly designed and powered boats have rather different functions. Apart from trim adjustment to compensate for variations in load, trim tabs speed up the transition from displacement cruising to planing. They can also be used to improve the ride in a seaway, and to compensate for any tendency to heel that may arise from uneven loading, such as a full or empty tank on the port or starboard side.

This potential for athwartships trimming has special advantages for motor yachts with a high superstructure which may be particularly affected by cross winds. A heeling motor yacht is unpleasant in its own right, but it also means that in choppy water the boat has a harder ride because the deadrise of the V-shaped underside is no longer bearing at its designed angle. Adjusting one trim tab allows you to straighten the

boat up again. Tab operation can either be electro-mechanical or electro-hydraulic, using rocker or lever switches or individual keys.

One thing trim tabs can't achieve is to increase the top speed, a false claim sometimes made for them by builders. However they do widen the range of economical planing and can reduce fuel consumption by up to 20%. You can see the reason for this because if a boat is already planing at 3000 revs, the engine will be drinking much less than if, without trim tabs, the boat could only plane at say 3800 revs.

The optimal setting for trim tabs can, again, only be established by trimming runs. At a variety of engine revs, you adjust the tab setting until you get to the highest speed and thus also the best trim. If the revs increase (a little) without your touching the throttle, thank the trim tabs. If they decrease, you're getting a negative effect. Once the boat has reached full

planing speed the trim tabs can only have a braking effect and accordingly increase consumption – so don't forget to set them back to zero as soon as they have done their job, unless they are needed to counteract heeling or a heavily loaded stern.

Less sophisticated versions of trim tabs are either fixed flaps, or the chocks which, instead of projecting from the transom, are built directly into the bottom of the boat from which they can be extended by a few degrees. These are not as effective or flexible as trim tabs, but they can sometimes be used to advantage to squeeze a little more speed from a displacement boat than its hull length permits, or to improve the performance of a planing boat which has been overloaded by heavy engines or equipment.

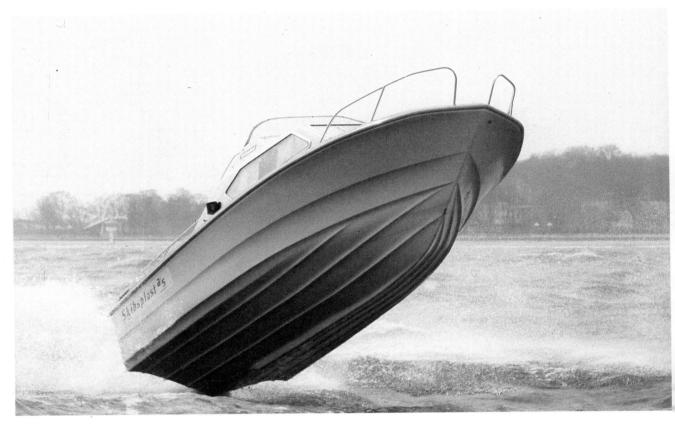

The higher they climb, the further they have to drop and thus the harder they smack down on the water. The forces to which the driver is exposed in the process are comparable to those acting on astronauts during the launch of their rocket. The way this boat is leaping is typical of a deep-V bottom, though. What we have here is a modern, modified-V hull shape. The driver has obviously hit a wave at the wrong speed or angle.

Dealing with hard-slamming boats

In certain boating circles, planing craft are considered to be hard slammers in a seaway but that, like so many things in life, is relative. However, it's true to say that as soon as you change from a displacement craft to a sporting, high-powered planing craft, you say good-bye to comfort. In rough seas all planing craft slam, only some do it more than others, and that's really what it's all about.

To some extent, you can see what to expect from a planing hull in rough seas just from looking at the shape of the bottom. The deeper the V the softer the ride, and the flatter the bottom the greater the tendency to slam. However, other factors are important as well. A short boat may fall into every 'hole' between waves and rise to every crest. Add just one metre to the length, and the same sea which gives the smaller boat a hard time may have very little effect on the larger. A ten metre, six tonne motor yacht will cut effortlessly through a chop which can make an inflatable leap high in the air.

Nevertheless every planing craft has its limits. Above a certain wave height

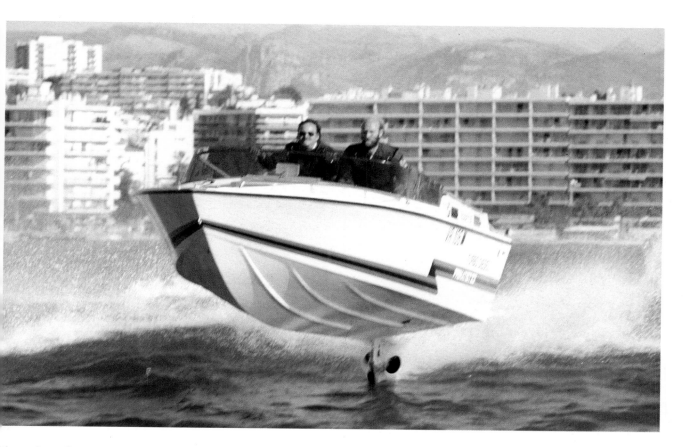

slamming for any normal driver becomes a physical torture and intolerable. Then, the only recourse is to the throttle back and cruise at displacement speed. But a little boat reaches its limits much sooner than a bit one. The only way of arriving at even approximately objective standards for the 'hardness' of a planing craft is by comparisons – as many as possible. Even in only moderate seas, lightweight planing craft – ranging from the open sports boat through the day cruiser up to the small motor yacht – tend to leap. Those that leap higher will slam harder, for the simple reason that they have further to fall. The

nose-in-the-air attitude when leaping is characteristic of boats with a constant V angle along the length of the hull. This sharp bottom shape lacks the necessary support at the stern, so there is no possibility of the air/water cushion developing which depresses the bow and eases the ride. If, on the other hand, the V becomes flatter towards the transom, as is usual these days, the bow will not lift so far and the drop (and therefore the slam) will be less. If, furthermore, such a boat is trimmed and powered correctly, its attitude in the air will be altogether more parallel to the water surface and its leaps are thus flatter. But helmsmen

The trim and power of this planing craft with a modified-V bottom are just right. The boat remains almost parallel to the surface as it leaps over the waves. The reduced dropping-distance is bound to mean softer landings. Some crews get a lot of fun from this kind of sportive planing.

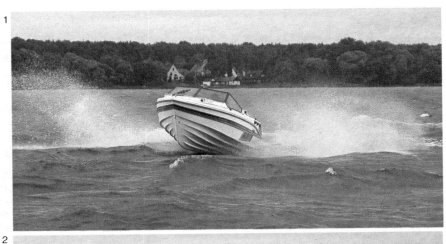

1

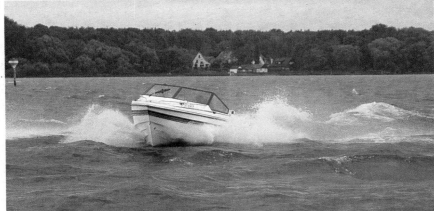

2

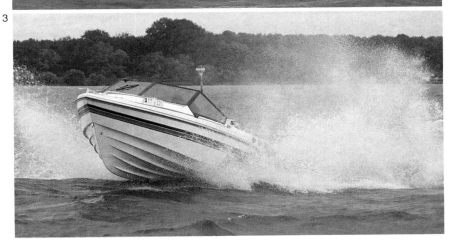

3

Leaps in the air are usually avoidable so long as you can steer a course at the right angle to the waves. With waves on the beam – as here – the boat will probably stick to the water at all times, provided you plane at a decent speed and don't timorously close the throttle. These three pictures show the behaviour of a smallish boat with waves more or less on the beam:

1 The boat is just riding on the crest of a wave arriving from the port side (slight heel to port) . . .

2 . . . it presses on with slightly lowered bows through the wave trough, the driver has turned into the waves a little . . .

3 . . . sits up on the next wave. The water is more choppy than it looks in the photograph; the height of the unpleasantly short waves of this large inland lake is about 0.4 metres – pretty rough seas for a smallish planing craft.

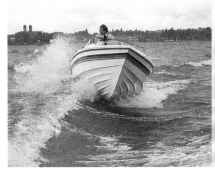

What can happen if you go too slowly in a beam sea? A shallow-draught planing craft is somewhat unstable running at displacement speeds. If a wave breaks against the side of the hull, the boat can be heeled strongly to leeward. At moments like this you need a firm hold of the wheel. The remedy, if that sort of thing keeps on happening, is to open the throttle and get on to the plane.

Not enough throttle – the boat topples off the wave crest and digs her bow in. You have to try and achieve a speed to enable the boat to leap over the wave trough and land on the next crest. Experienced drivers manage to keep up this wave-hopping over long distances.

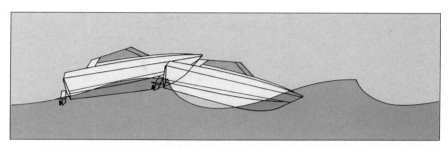

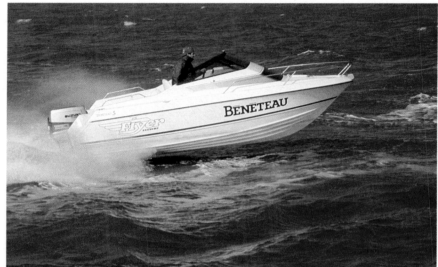

A well driven and trimmed boat, leaping from wave to wave with only the aft part of the hull immersed. Since the contact point has moved well back from where the driver sits, the shocks there are no longer so hard. Seeing this boat is a reminder that a boat with an outboard is no less seaworthy than one with an inboard engine. On the other side of the Atlantic, most boats up to and beyond day-cruiser size have outboard engines, even those for use in coastal waters.

beware. If, on immersion after a leap, the boat is struck by a cross wave, things can get very nasty for a careless driver and the boat may be knocked off course harshly. Of course you can always throttle back in a rough sea. That immediately puts an end to those sporting leaps in the air and the slamming, but also reduces much of the fun in motor boating.

In any case, planing over rough seas is not pure masochism. Planing craft cruising slowly at displacement speeds run extremely uneconomically. Considered from that point of view, the wish to carry on planing for as long as possible is perfectly understandable. Sometimes, indeed, running 'softly' – again, relatively – can be a matter of having the courage to push the throttle further forward. When planing slowly, many boats have the centre of immersion pretty far forward, usually just about where the driver sits. Slams are usually hardest at that point, which is why the most sought-after seats in a planing craft are usually aft where the slamming is least. As soon as you accelerate, the point of immersion moves aft and you get the apparent paradox that, though the increase in speed makes the water 'harder', for the driver and co-driver the boat now seems to be running more smoothly or agreeably. In these circumstances, with the boat riding only on its prop and its 'buttocks', it's the after seats which are pretty uncomfortable.

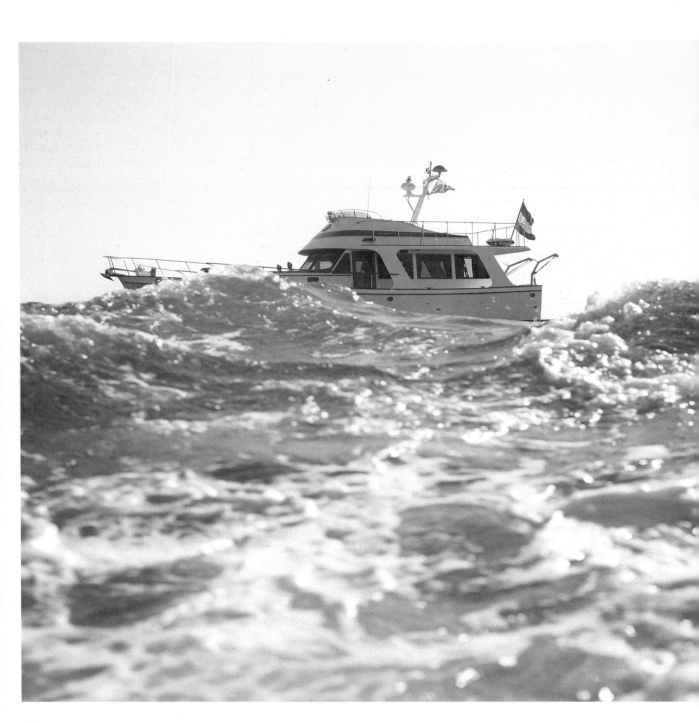

Motor boats in rough water

What is 'rough water' for a motor boat? Using wind strength as a guide to sea conditions, which is the common practice, actually doesn't make a lot of sense, because what causes trouble for the motor boat is what the wind produces (the waves) and for a given wind strength these can vary quite considerably. Much depends, for example, on whether wind and current are in opposition, which can steepen the waves into evil, short little monsters; and whether you are in deep or shallow water, or shielded by land, which can provide effective shelter for several miles out to sea. It is quite possible to be still planing in a 26 foot boat in a force 7 wind under the shelter of the coast, but be unable to do so in force 4–5 further offshore.

To be ploughing through really rough seas is, in any case, a miserable and dangerous business and you are

Left: Running before a sea. This sort of wave, of more than freeboard height and about the same length as the boat, is most unpleasant.

well advised to stay at home in that sort of weather. But it could nevertheless happen that you get caught out in more than you had bargained for or than the weather forecast had indicated. That's when it's useful to know what to do and what your boat will stand. In fact if a motor yacht is really 'seagoing' it can, with an experienced hand on the wheel and throttle, get through almost any kind of weather so long as the engines keep going. Undoubtedly, boats are sold and bought as 'seagoing' which reach their absolute limit in conditions associated with winds of force 6 or 7. On the other hand, the definition of seagoing given by one well-known builder of large fast motor yachts is: 'Able at least to stay afloat in a storm and a corresponding sea. To be able to reach port safely and, preferably, to reach the intended destination more or less according to schedule, with minimal disagreeable motion on board.' Disagreeable conditions for a motor boat occur when the relationship between boat length and wave length is wrong. An awkward sea for most hulls is one

with a wave length of between one and two boat lengths and a height about the same as the freeboard. When running before such a sea it's usually very difficult to keep the boat on course. From about three boat lengths upwards it can still be awkward, but not really particularly dangerous. However, when thinking about the behaviour and control of motor boats in rough seas, it is again necessary to distinguish between displacement and planing hulls.

Heading into the sea with a motor yacht often means continual work with the throttle:
1 Increase power to run up the slope of the wave and then throttle back as soon as the bow projects above the crest to prevent the propeller thrashing the air at high revs as the boat pitches (2) into the trough. Open the throttle a bit running down the slope, and at the bottom of the trough open her up again for a charge up the next slope.

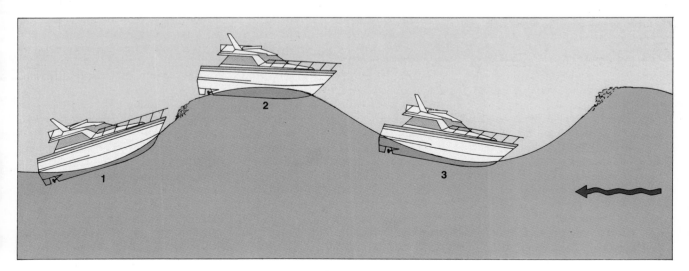

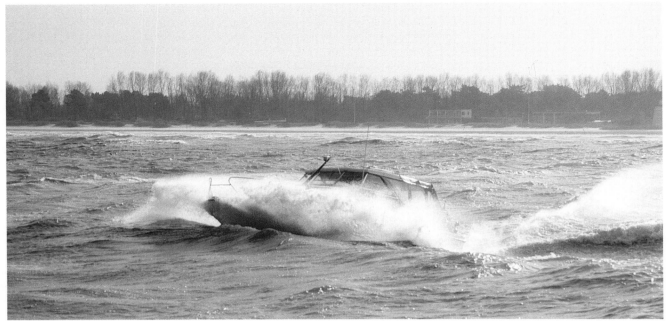

A heavy ground swell is often worse than it looks. This boat is crashing slap into a wave too fast. It's going to be wet on deck and the windscreen wiper is going to have to work overtime.

Displacement craft in heavy seas

Round bilge displacement craft have a tendency to roll and pitch ominously in seas of a certain shape and period. This occurs when the natural frequency of the boat's motions – which after all are also oscillations – corresponds precisely to that of the seas. This results in an unpleasant build-up of motion which is preventable only to some extent. Moving weights (portable equipment, etc) from the axis of rotation of the motion (ie from amidships) nearer to the ends (ie forward or aft) lengthens the period of the motion. Conversely, the period can be shortened by re-stowing heavy weights from the ends amidships.

When running before wind and waves, it's not long before most displacement craft start becoming a handful. The helmsman has to keep watching like a hawk to avoid the risk of broaching-to. Practical tests with a range of boats have shown that they must not run at more than about 5.5 km/h (3 kn) in heavy following seas to stay roughly on course. Clearly, it will not always be possible to slow down that far. The tactic of streaming lines astern to provide a towing resistance is usually of dubious value. For one thing there is a danger that just when the boat should be free to rise to a sea, the stern is held down by the lines. Propellers are also very vulnerable to towing lines, especially when a wave is at the point of overtaking the boat.

Running beam-on to wind and sea is also very nerve racking. A strongly rounded bilge acts like the rockers of a rocking horse, rolling and reeling the hull from side to side, and the boat can heel over so far that the leeward gunwale digs in deep and scoops a sizeable amount of water into the cockpit as the boat rights again. Although the skipper may become accustomed to this motion, his crew may have more difficulty with their apprehensions and seasickness.

You will really only find out with your own boat in what sort of sea states you will have to head slowly into the weather to make the only really safe course. Motoring head-to, or nearly head-to, sea will bring a lot of spray but is inherently less dangerous. The trick is to set the throttle so that the bow can just climb the waves without difficulty. If you go even a little too fast, the bow will not rise

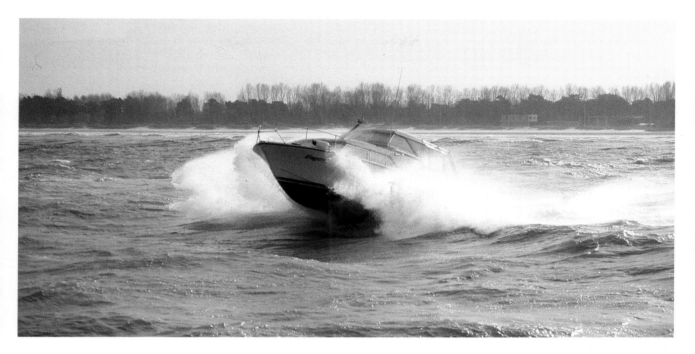

above the crest of the wave but drive through it instead. The seas then breaking over the boat could, under certain circumstances, break the windows and fill the saloon. If, on the other hand, the boat is inclined to undercut the waves or to pitch heavily, you have to head into the sea at an angle – usually between 30° and 40°, but no more than necessary to stop the bow undercutting. Steering can then become really hard work because the boat keeps trying to yaw. In weather like this, much depends on the skill of the helmsman. The beginner, as soon as the boat starts to yaw, tends to apply heavy rudder to bring it back on course. He will end up by swinging the wheel continuously and in a little while will become extremely tired. An experienced helmsman, on the other hand, allows the boat a degree of yaw and then slowly brings it back on course with a small amount of rudder.

Some helmsmen almost seem to have a sixth sense for the sea, which is something you can't really learn. This is the ability to assess beforehand, from the look of a wave, how strongly it will affect the boat and her course. Such a helmsman applies opposite rudder in advance, gently and precisely to anticipate the effect of the wave and take the sting out of it.

A motor yacht that gets into heavy weather needs sea room to windward to be able to head into the wind. Adopting this tactic, the yacht may still be moving ahead at 2 or 3 knots. The impression – and this is a widespread fallacy – that the boat is doing no more than countering the approaching seas, can be deceptive. The waves are not a flowing current but just a stationary up-and-down motion.

In extreme conditions, there are displacement craft which, even when

When powering through a wave, care must be taken not to shoot out too far beyond it (throttle back in good time). This is typical rough-water behaviour of a planing or a semi-displacement craft. The bow splits the waves and brushes them aside.

heading into the sea, ship so much water that there is the risk of damage to the superstructure. Of course there may not be enough power to make any headway at all against the heavy seas. The next tactic to consider is to stop the engine and effectively leave the boat to ride to the elements. The boat may end up heading about halfway into the wind and will roll heavily with the waves, but should not ship much water. Like that you can, albeit with a considerably distressed stomach, ride out almost any storm provided the hull can stand it. In that situation, the boat needs considerable sea room to leeward, so that it can drift safely in open water.

Planing craft in heavy seas

Planing craft – and this includes superfast displacement craft – by virtue of their flat bottom and strong deadrise don't build up a roll. Their so-called roll period is too short and doesn't fit the wave period of a wind-generated sea of any strength. Even nowadays, the opinion is widespread that planing craft cannot run before wind and sea. On the contrary, they just need to be driven differently and call for speedier reactions. The deeper the V of the bottom, the better their course stability when running before a sea.

The ratio of boat to wave length, which is so critical for displacement craft, provides fewer problems for planing craft. You can usually trump such a wave's tricks by adjusting your

speed. All that's needed is the courage to push down the throttle. Then the boat leaps over the wave troughs and only sets its stern down on the crests. Of course, unless you react swiftly and skilfully with the throttle, this type of manoeuvre doesn't always succeed. Because wave spacing isn't 'standard', it's quite easy to come down precisely between two waves and run the bow slap into the next advancing slope. The thought of having to go faster when you're already pounding along may well be alarming if you've never driven a planing craft in rough seas, but once you get used to the idea it's surprising how effectively the boat can cope with what's thrown at it. Of course there comes a point where even the most seaworthy of planing craft have to slow down and travel at displacement speed.

When cruising beam-on to rough seas, planing craft often perform much better than displacement boats. Perhaps surprisingly, this point of cruising can be faster and decidedly more pleasant than any other course. The offshore racers are well aware of

this and make use of it. A planing craft will, during such a ride, give its crew a much greater feeling of security than a displacement craft. When running before a heavy sea the throttle is more use in a planing craft than the rudder. You have to try to adjust your speed to match the progress of the waves. If you succeed, you will motor up and down quite impressive waves with a rocking motion that is almost pleasant.

The one really critical situation is over-running a wave crest by going too fast and then roaring down into the trough. On the leading slope of the wave the boat, because of its own force of gravity, speeds up anyway. If you are trying to motor fast as well, the bow may be unable to cope with the build up of water ahead of it. The bow digs in, the boat stops suddenly,

This is an extreme example of what can happen if you're going too fast in a following wind and sea and find yourself overtaking the waves. Since most motor yachts are a bit top-heavy, there is a risk of pitchpoling.

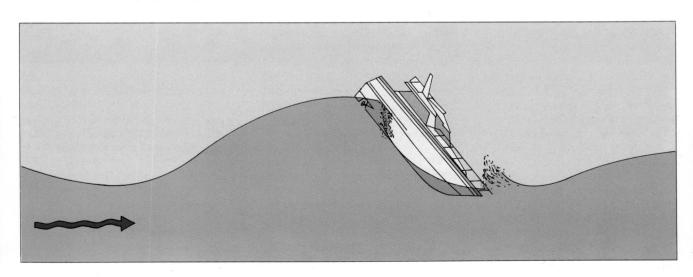

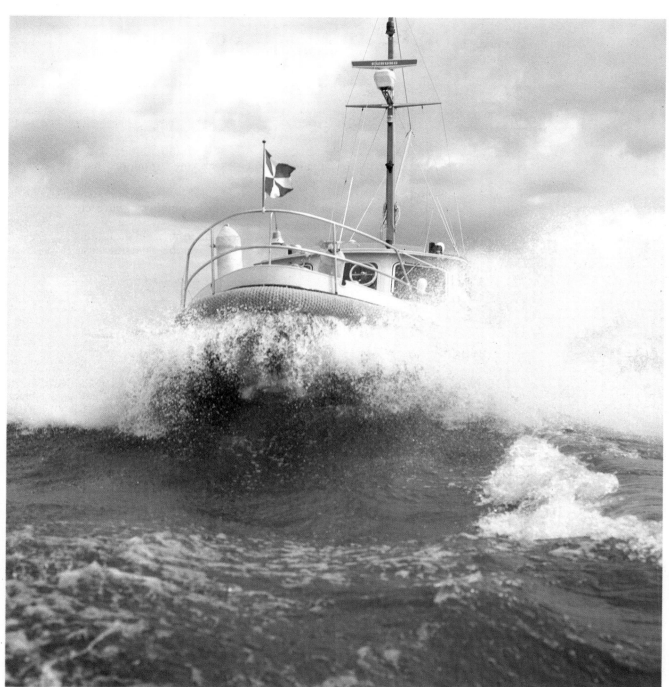

A typical displacement craft, shovelling her way through a heavy sea.

the stern is lifted up by the following sea, and the whole boat could be in danger of pitchpoling, stern over bow. This danger exists in precisely the same way for displacement craft.

On the other hand, a planing craft is not so prone to broaching-to before a following sea. Close the throttle, and the next wave should run harmlessly through under the boat. But it would be a wrong move to haul the throttle back just as the bow begins to get dug-in in the trough of the wave. The stern would just be dragged around more violently. If this should happen, the best tactic is to use only a little throttle, but a good kick of the rudder to turn back on to your initial course, preferably, watching out for a series of low waves to do it. During the climb up a wave slope you can then resume your old speed.

If a particularly steep and impressive breaker comes roaring up astern, it would be wrong to slow down abruptly or indeed stop. The boat's own stern wave would just become superimposed on the approaching rogue, this would catch up with the boat and then break dangerously over the stern. It is best to keep going, but if possible at a slower speed than the wave moving forwards. What you have to resist is the temptation to try to stay on top of a wave crest. A momentary inattention here and you run a significant risk of capsize. Whenever you have to slow the boat down, remember that a slow-running propeller achieves this better than one which is stopped altogether.

Only boats with a guaranteed speed of about 40 km/h, and therefore able to match wave speeds, can be ridden on the back of a ground swell over a bar into a river mouth or harbour. You have to juggle with the throttle so that the boat neither climbs onto the crest nor drops astern into the trough. Of course it is safer not to get mixed up with a ground swell at all. If you do have to, watch the pattern of the seas as you approach the bar, then try to catch a series of smaller-than-average waves. You then head the boat on course and, as soon as these waves overtake you, accelerate to match their speed and try to keep in the trough behind the leading wave. There, the water is usually relatively smooth. But the driver has to maintain concentration, since he must neither overtake the wave ahead nor be overtaken by the one astern. It is a spectacular manoeuvre for anyone watching – and for the others in the boat.

A mostly decked-over motor cruiser with high freeboard should be able to get home, perhaps travelling slowly at displacement speed, under most sea conditions that can arise in coastal waters. A day cruiser with a large cockpit isn't quite so seaworthy. Heading into the weather can be difficult in a short, steep sea if the length of the boat doesn't quite 'fit'. Digging her bow in is then a real danger. A single wave washing 'green' over foredeck and windscreen can be enough to fill the cockpit to the gunwales. For anyone who has been through this it will have been a frightening experience. At that moment one is totally helpless – no assistance can be had from either rudder or throttle – and all one can do is trust to the boat's advertised unsinkability.

If there is reason to fear that the boat may dig in when running at displacement speed, accelerate at once to something just short of planing speed, which should bring the bows well up out of the water. Driven thus, the risk of digging in is much reduced. The driver of a planing craft is in the fortunate position of being able to influence the angle at which his boat faces the sea. The displacement craft driver can't do this. He has to put up with each sea as it comes.

If things get really bad you can always try stopping the engine and letting the boat cope naturally with the seas. Your rolling motion will still be less unpleasant for the crew than that of a displacement craft. It can be comforting to appreciate this, and realise that a planing boat can usually ride things out in the event of an engine failure.

Finally, on the question of the relative seaworthiness of displacement and planing boats, it cannot be denied that speed can contribute greatly to safety at sea. If the weather deteriorates unexpectedly you will certainly appreciate a 20 knot cruising speed and the ability to reach the nearest harbour before freshening winds turn a pleasant trip into a fight for survival. If you are caught out though, remember that wind and rough seas have a marked effect on fuel consumption, sometimes increasing it by up to 100%. You can therefore find yourself with not enough fuel to reach a safe haven. If the weather and sea conditions force you to slow down in a twin-engined boat you can reduce fuel consumption drastically by running on one engine only. This straightaway halves the consumption. If you can't switch between tanks you will have to run the starboard and port engines alternately.

Driving on rivers and in currents

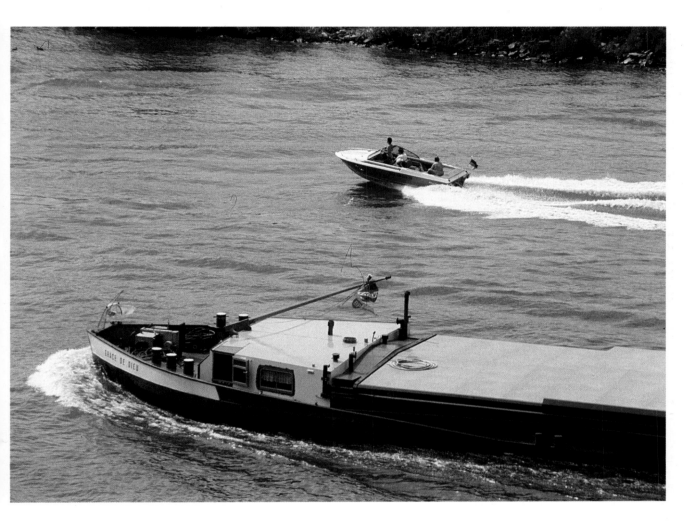

Tidal waters or river currents significantly influence the way you drive. A following current increases the boat's speed by its own speed, while an opposing current slows you down correspondingly. An insufficiently powered boat may well be unable to breast a strong tide or current. The more slowly the boat is moving, the greater the influence of the current – something you have to take into account when stopping or berthing.

Steering by eye in a strong current is a knack which comes with practice. You have to get used to predicting, more or less instinctively, the combined effect of the forward motion of the boat and the run of the stream, whether this is setting crosswise, acting with, or acting against the boat. A directly following or opposing tide or current doesn't divert the boat from its track at all, whereas sideways drift is greatest with the tide or current on the beam, ie setting at right-angles to your track.

If you are steering for a distant mark by eye and there is a current setting across your course, you'll end up by following a curved track (as with route numbers 1 and 3 on page 107). If, however, you steer a corrected course to allow for the cross-set, the boat should end up by following a straight track (as with route number 2), even though the bow will be

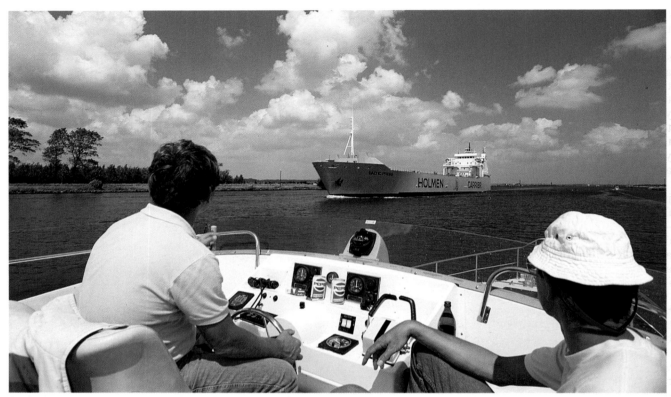

Always keep a good lookout. You usually get a much better view of the traffic from the flybridge than from the helming position in the saloon.

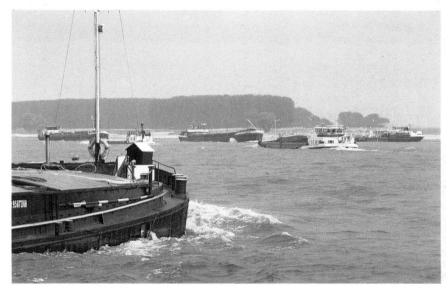

Who is going which way? A helmsman unused to inland waterways with heavy traffic may well be apprehensive when faced with a line of jostling barges.

continually pointing off to one side of the mark you are aiming for.

A useful trick for assessing your sideways drift is to line up two marks ashore ahead or astern and watch how their relative position changes. If the two marks stay exactly in line, then you are actually moving directly towards (or away from) them, even though, because of the cross-current, your bow will not be pointing directly at the transit.

The strength of the current can be judged from the inclination of floating fairway markers – buoys and suchlike – and the trail of eddies which form down-stream from them. However, to assess the actual speed of a current accurately from these indicators requires a great deal of experience.

On large navigable rivers, seagoing sailors lacking experience in inland cruising may well be puzzled by the behaviour of barges and cargo vessels which repeatedly cut across the fairway. However there are usually good reasons for this. In fairly sharp bends, the main flow of a river swings from one bank to the other, the current running significantly faster near the outside of the bends. Professional skippers make full use of this. When going upstream, they take the path of least resistance – the inside of the bend. Going downstream, on the

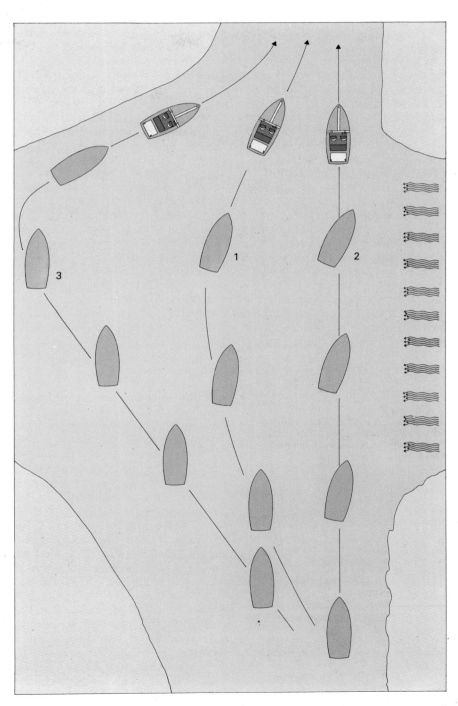

Passing a cross-current
1 Attempting to maintain a steady course will produce a curved track over the ground.
2 To prevent this you have to head slightly into the cross-current, depending on its strength.
3 It can be more economical just to let the cross-current push you sideways and then head up again in the slower stream near the bank – even if it is a bit further.

other hand, they exploit the faster running current on the outside of the bends. Yachts have to keep a sharp eye on this 'pendulum' progress of barges from bank to bank, especially if they are travelling in the opposite direction. Otherwise it could easily happen that you suddenly find yourself under the bow of a large barge which has suddenly appeared like a ghost from behind the stern of the vessel ahead, and is now heading straight for you.

Yacht skippers with river experience also make use of the current. Since it is usually strongest where the water is deep, towards the middle of the river, that's where they try to stay when going downstream. Going upstream, on the other hand, it is often best to stick to the shallower water near the bank, thereby saving both fuel and time. Unfortunately,

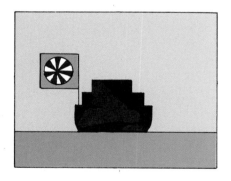

On large Continental rivers, vessels heading upstream give way to vessels coming downstream, because the latter are less manoeuvrable. Usually, both keep to the right and pass port-to-port. However, if the vessel heading upstream wants the one going down to pass to *starboard*, this is indicated by a light blue flag on her starboard side, or a light blue panel with a quick flashing white light.

especially on the European waterways, you rarely have a river to yourself. To port perhaps a tug and tow, to starboard two motor vessels overtaking one another, ahead maybe two barges meeting, with wash from ahead, astern and abeam crossing unpleasantly. You can also meet eddies and cross-currents – sometimes powerful enough to give you some pretty uncomfortable moments. It can also be dangerous to find yourself between two large freighters passing or overtaking one another close together. Between such 'fatties' not only do you get a horrible chop, quite annoying enough by itself, but also a powerful suction which can be enough for a small, low powered boat to broach-to or be forced against the side of one of the larger vessels.

Passing and overtaking

Where freighters are passing each other, it's best to keep well back. Drop astern from the ship steaming ahead of you, far enough for the one coming the other way to be able to see your boat throughout the manoeuvre. There is a simple rule of thumb here: as long as you can see his steering position from your own helming position, he will also be able to see you. If you yourself want to overtake, the first thing to make sure is that you can get past before the next bend. Only overtake if you have a clear view of at least one kilometre of the river, so never in loops or ahead of bends. Obviously when overtaking or passing you leave a reasonable gap – 10 metres at least – to stay clear of the suction zone. This is particularly pronounced over the larger ship's forward quarter, and in the wake immediately astern.

A displacement motor craft will usually be slower than a freighter, and therefore will frequently be the overtaken vessel. You pull over to one side, away from the ship's course as far as possible, to avoid the worst of the suction and wash. In a displacement yacht, you will also have to accept having to trail along for hours behind a slow tug and tow because you probably won't have enough speed to struggle past safely. This can be very frustrating on busy rivers and canals.

In a planing craft, you will probably be able to overtake slower merchant vessels more easily. Bow and stern waves are best crossed at an angle of about 80°. In between the two, there is usually a system of smaller waves, which can be cut more acutely to avoid getting too close to the ship and its suction zone. When overtaking, you should stay inside the stern wave until you're about 10 metres from the stern, then open the throttle and cut through it at an angle. But you mustn't take the bow or stern waves at too high a speed. They may look harmless as they come rolling along but they are often higher and more powerful than you imagine. Novices have great difficulty in assessing the power and height of a wave from a big ship correctly. The powerful blows which the boat and her crew may receive, and for which they are often not prepared, could fling an unsuspecting crew dangerously across the cockpit and break a lot of china in the galley. The crew in a small open boat should, as a matter of course, get into the habit of holding on to the grab handle or some other secure handhold. However, it would be equally wrong to take fright at the sight of the impressive looking bow wave of a big ship and slow down from planing to displacement speed. This can lead to

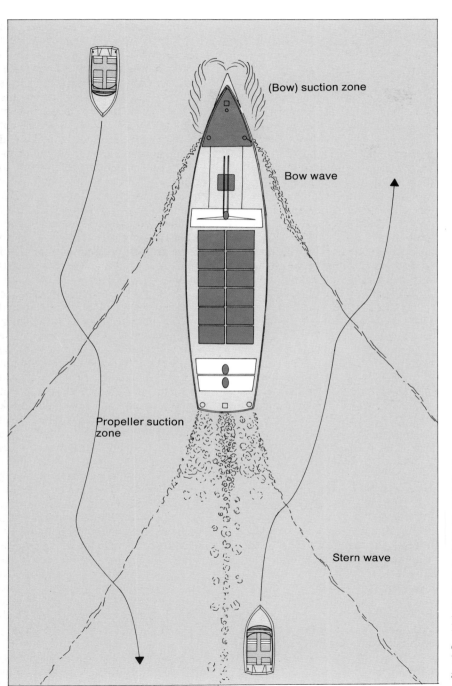

(Bow) suction zone

Bow wave

Propeller suction zone

Stern wave

Crossing bow and stern waves in either direction

When meeting a barge, steer clear far enough to be able to cross the bow wave roughly at right angles. In the calm water zone between the barge's bow and stern wave, turn back on to a parallel course to stay clear of the suction effect of the prop as you cross the stern wave.

When overtaking, again steer clear of the suction effect of the prop and cross the stern wave roughly at right angles. Then steer away from the barge to avoid getting into the suction zone near her bow.

the bow digging in and, at least in an open boat, shipping a lot of water into the cockpit. The right way for small boats to handle this situation is to approach the wash at moderate planing speed, throttle back on the crest to stop the boat overshooting, and accelerate again as soon as you start down the back slope. Alternatively you can carry out the operation slowly, at displacement speed. Then you don't have to juggle with the throttle at all. When overtaking, however, that slow rate of progress will not be enough to get you across the wash and safely past the ship.

A sharp turn going downstream – a typical small river port on the Continental waterways (Oberwinter on the Rhine). The entrance narrows to a bottleneck facing downstream, and it's usually best to enter fairly quickly to cope with the backwash off the breakwater.

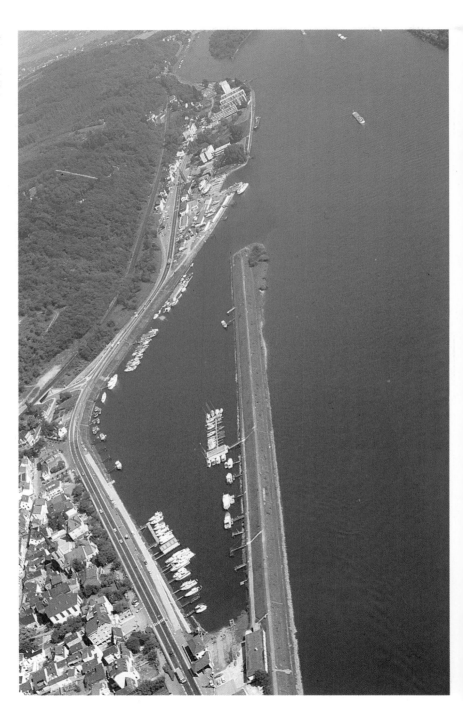

River ports – entering and leaving

River ports usually have to be shared with cargo vessels and other commercial traffic. Yacht harbours or marinas on their own are fairly rare.

On the European waterways, smallish river ports often have a protective wall parallel to the river bank, with the narrow entrance pointing downstream. When entering, it's best to keep close to the pierhead, because sometimes there is a mudbank lurking off the riverbank. If the river current is fast, there will probably be a pretty strong back eddy in the entrance. Behind the pierhead you may meet whirlpools and eddies, well able to push a low-powered boat out of control. Before leaving a busy river port, look out for ships about to enter, which might suddenly appear 'round the corner'.

In some ports, certain sound signals are obligatory for merchant vessels, and sometimes yachts on leaving.

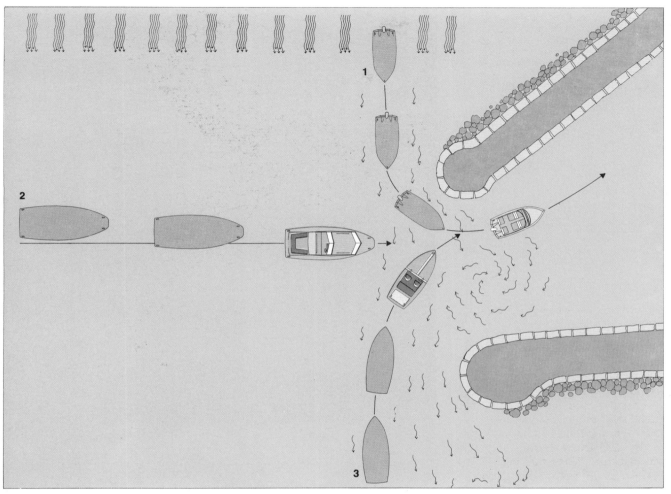

Negotiating a narrow entrance

1 With the current: Because of the following stream, you arrive quite quickly but your boat doesn't respond particularly well to the rudder. The moment for turning-in has to be judged exactly right if you're not to shoot past the entrance.

2 Across the current: This is when the effect of the current is most noticeable, so you have to keep well upstream on the approach. You must adopt similar tactics when manoeuvring across the current between bridge supports and suchlike.

3 Against the current: Don't start turning until you're in the upstream part of the entrance.

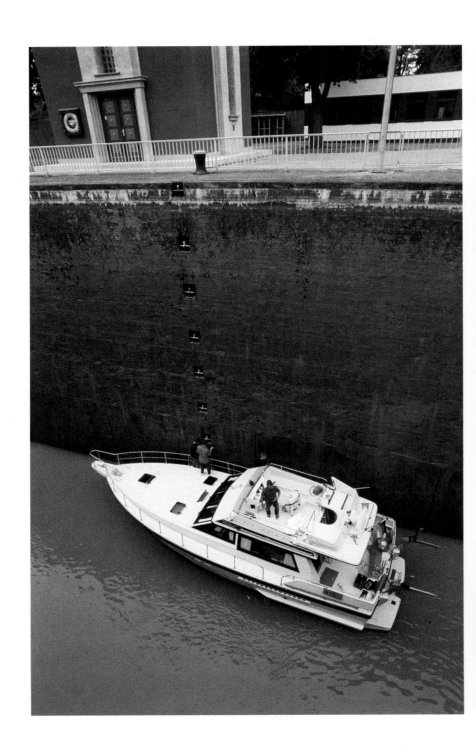

Locks

There are all kinds of locks: single, twin, or multi-chamber locks; lifting, hinged, and sliding-gate locks, or locks with submersible gates. Tidal harbour lock gates retain the water in a basin over the low tide period to prevent the vessels in the basin from drying out. For this reason their opening times are usually limited to a couple of hours either side of high water. Entry and exit are often regulated by traffic lights on one or both sides of the lock chamber. This can be confusing the first time, with white, green, and red lights flashing in front of you without your knowing what they mean. And, what is even more confusing, the meaning of the light signals is quite likely to differ from harbour to harbour.

When approaching a lock you sometimes find barges or cargo vessels waiting in the outer port area. Don't try to jump the queue ahead of these ships, but hold well back until it becomes clear whether they or you are expected to enter the lock first. If the wait looks like being protracted, go alongside a quay or another boat and keep an eye on events.

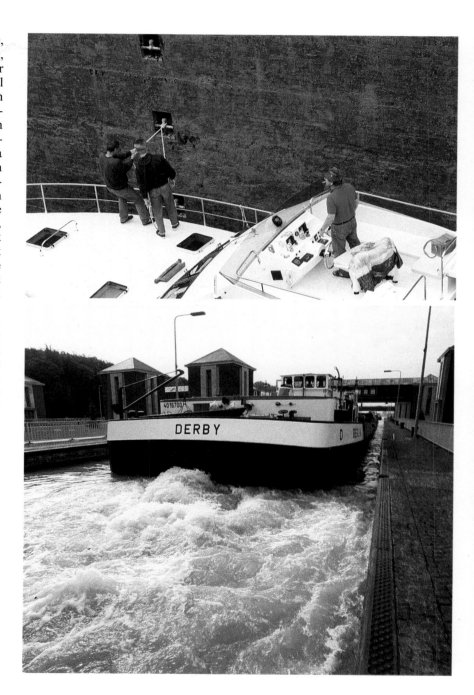

Left and above right: Rig a slip rope to one of the bollards set in the chamber wall, remembering to move it in time as the water level changes. Don't let the bow or stern sheer away from the lock chamber wall.

Right: That's what it looks like when one of those large barges gets under way inside a lock – an impressive wash from the propeller. Small boats should wait until things quieten down before leaving.

Under no circumstances should you enter an open lock without instructions. Merchant shipping has absolute priority, unless the lock-keeper prefers to take yachts in first. Furthermore, small yachts are not usually locked through singly; there have to be enough yachts waiting to be locked 'en masse'. Sometimes there may be special pleasure craft locks alongside the main shipping locks. Always follow the lock-keeper's instructions carefully.

You should already have rigged a generous number of fenders while waiting, and laid out the mooring warps ready forward and aft. When entering the lock basin it's advisable to keep a respectful distance from the last cargo vessel, otherwise you may find yourself caught up in its propeller wash and carried out of control. The best way of making fast depends on the layout of the lock, and also on how it is flooded and pumped out.

Some locks are peaceful, so that even largish yachts can be held securely by hand. Others are extremely turbulent. There are locks where the water is reused, filled from a storage basin alongside, and emptied into that again. The berths nearest the inlets and outlets can be pretty uncomfortable because of the strong eddies generated, which tug at your warps.

Locks can be pretty daunting structures with their high wet walls covered in green slime, which sometimes have to be climbed by means of slippery iron ladders to get the lines to the top.

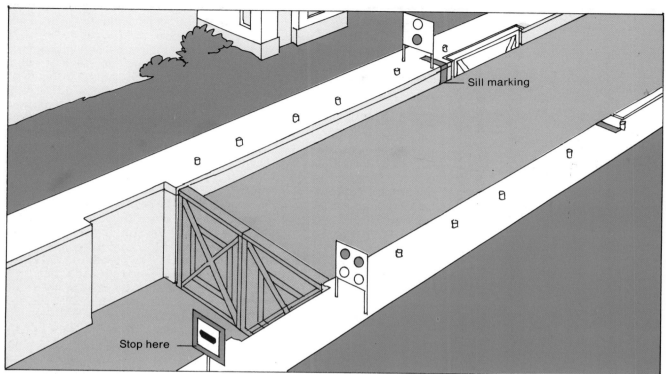

Sill marking

Stop here

Traffic light rules for locks

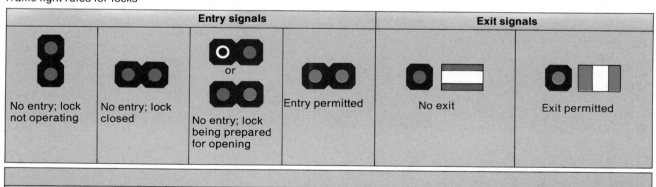

Entry signals				Exit signals	
No entry; lock not operating	No entry; lock closed	No entry; lock being prepared for opening	Entry permitted	No exit	Exit permitted

Lh steady, rh flashing: use rh lock chamber

Rh steady, lh flashing: use lh lock chamber

Both lights steady: await instructions for entry

Both lights flashing: either lock chamber may be used

115

If you're lucky, someone on the lockside will take your warps. Otherwise you have to send a crew member up a ladder to look for a suitable bollard, ring or whatever the lock has to offer. Whether you're going up or down, all lines should be 'slipped' ideally so that they can be cast off at any time and moved to the next higher or lower bollard. With slipped mooring lines, the end of the rope which is placed around the lock bollard should not have a bowline or spliced eye, which could easily catch on something or become inextricably jammed behind a ring. Simplest are the locks

with floating pontoons, so that you can come alongside and make fast normally, without worrying about tending warps as you rise or fall.

To come alongside a large vessel in a lock is not as clever as it might seem at first sight, and isn't usually popular either. You can get into pretty serious trouble if a large barge or ship which has been carelessly secured starts to swing in the lock eddies or when getting under way. It can also happen that two barges on either side of the chamber get under way almost simultaneously, dramatically reducing the gap between them. A relatively fragile

yacht in this position would be in a dangerous situation.

When being lowered you have to be careful not to get your boat caught on top of the lock sill. White or yellow marks on the walls indicate (but by no means always!) how far this sill projects into the chamber. In locks with sheet piling walls, fenders are prone to jam in the recesses, and the projecting steel boltheads can make a nasty mess of a yacht's topside if you are not well fendered.

Before leaving a lock, the warps should be kept fast until larger vessels ahead have left and the wash has calmed down a bit. To get steerage way, well-laden barges have to use plenty of power, and the turbulence this causes can be dangerous for a small boat. The beamier the vessel ahead, the more carefully it needs to be treated.

Finally a tip. Lock walls are not only wet and slimey but also extraordinarily dirty and usually pretty rough as well. If you have to lock frequently and like to keep your warps clean, you ought to acquire a couple of cheap, stout, hemp or polypropylene lines for that purpose alone. A few old trailer or caravan tyres sewn into sailcloth save wear and tear on your expensive yacht fenders.

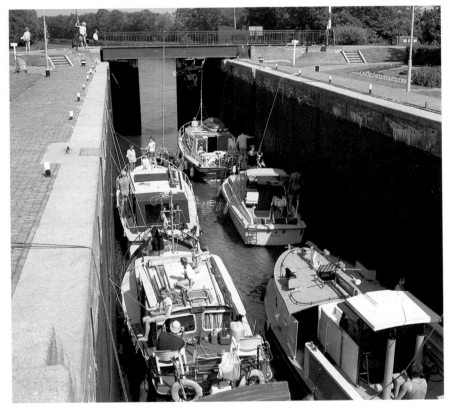

Locks can sometimes be companionable places, as this picture shows.

Towing and being towed

If your engine breaks down you are in a tricky situation, whether this happens at sea or on inland waters. You are fortunate if you find someone quickly to tow you into the nearest harbour or out of the fairway. On lengthy river journeys there's sometimes the opportunity of a tow offered by a barge, particularly if you have insufficient power to cope with the current.

If you are going to do the towing, you should get as close as possible to the boat you are helping; go into neutral and accept their line in the cockpit. If this is thrown short and flops into the water between the boats, don't engage gear again until the rope has been retrieved, otherwise it may foul your prop and immobilise your own boat as well. Where there is a current or tide, try to approach against the current because it's better for manoeuvring. Towing puts a heavy strain on cleats or bollards so, if possible, the load should be spread over several attachment points. Ideally, the pull of the two should be along the centreline of the boat. If you don't have an appropriate fitting on the centreline aft, it makes sense to fasten the tow line to the two stern cleats using a bridle made up from one of your warps. That arrangement is a must if the tow is a larger or heavier boat than yours.

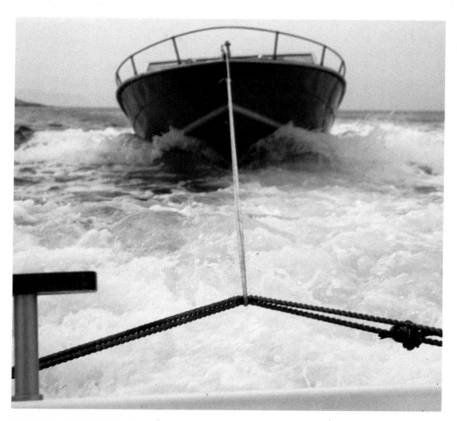

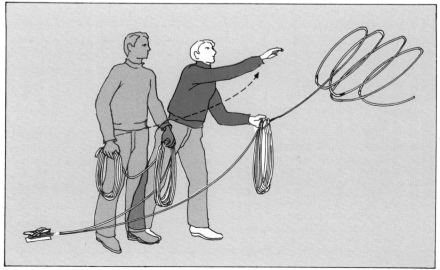

Passing a line: First coil the line, then take about a third of the coils in the throwing hand, aim for a point just behind the man on the shore, and throw with a sweeping upward movement. The coils open out in the air, and your other hand simultaneously feeds out the rest of the line.

Smallish boats requiring a tow should secure the tow-line to a stempost if possible, which is usually better able to stand the strain than a bow cleat. Reaching the stempost or cleat across the foredeck of a small boat is often difficult, so you should get into the habit of fastening a stout line to it before starting any trip. This can be used variously as a painter, warp or securing point for a tow line.

When the tow line has been secured aboard both boats, start slowly so that the full pull comes on only gradually, not with a jerk. Barge skippers in a hurry, but prepared to give a pleasure craft a lift, understandably don't want to lose a lot of time doing so, and thus slow down only a little. You should approach them from astern, leaving a gap large enough for safety (suction!). As soon as you are abreast the stern of the barge, throw the tow line across and drop back as soon as it has been safely caught, paying the line out hand over hand to its full length. First belay it securely, because you won't be able

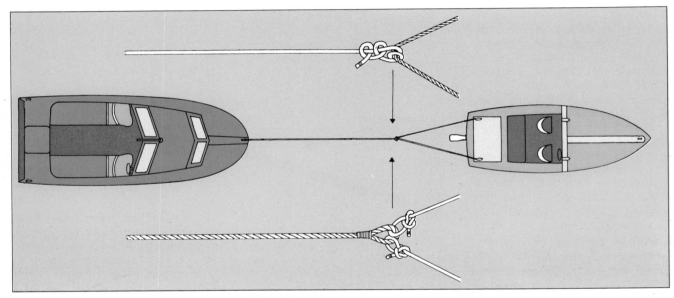

Above: Spreading the load: To avoid overloading one cleat, and to improve manoeuvrability, spread the load from the tow-line to both stern cleats by using a bridle. Here are two ways of making up a temporary bridle and connecting it to the tow-line.

Right: With heavy motor yachts you can use the anchor chain to take some of the tensile strain of the towing cable. Stoppers hooked into the chain and taken to the bow cleats take some of the load off the anchor winch. However the length of chain run out should not be more than about half that of the boat. Use a pin or lashing to hold the chain down in the bow roller and prevent it from jumping out under a sideways pull.

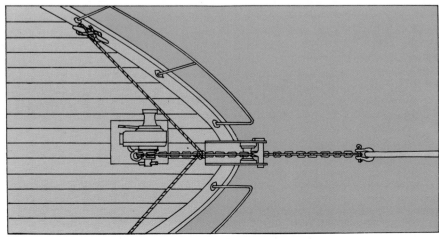

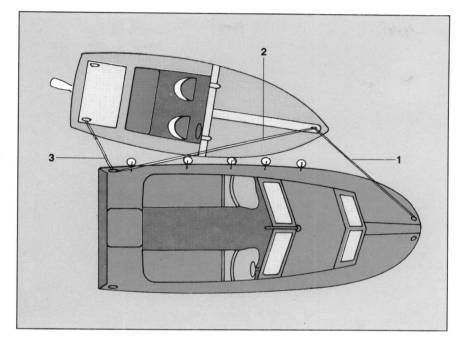

Towing alongside: If the 'tug' is substantially smaller than the boat to be towed, it should be secured as far aft as possible and angled slightly bows-in. This is the only arrangement which, with the rudder angled slightly outwards, allows a reasonably straight course to be steered. The tug's angle is controlled by the bow (1) and stern (3) lines; the tow-line proper is the tug's spring (2) which takes the main pulling strain.

to do that once the strain comes on. Look lively as well. Most barge skippers are in the habit of going full ahead as soon as their end of the line is secured, regardless of whether or not you have paid it out fully at your end. Particularly when getting under way, but also as a general rule, the crew of both boats should keep well clear of the tow rope; if it should part the whiplash can be dangerous.

At sea and in waters where traffic density permits this, you should pay out enough line so that it hangs down in a slight bight. This introduces some elasticity in the tow to help prevent snubbing and violent jerks on cleats and other fittings.

Where both tug and tow are motor boats, the towing speed will present no problems for either. The situation is very different, though, if you are being towed behind a barge, or perhaps a

large fishing boat. Displacement craft towed at more than their hull speed run the risk of broaching-to, capsizing, or suffering damage to their hull and fittings. A large wave builds up around the bow, and should this coincide with a steep sea in choppy conditions, a displacement craft being towed too fast can dig in and, in extreme cases, fill with water and sink.

When you've got your tow to its destination, once again you have to take care that the line cast off doesn't foul your prop. If the line belongs to the other boat, you should throw it well clear, preferably back on his foredeck. If the rope is your own, you should only gather it in with your engine out of gear.

In narrow fairways, harbour areas and when locking, towing alongside is recommended, as in the diagram above. If the 'tug' has a single screw,

you take the boat to be towed on the side towards which the prop turns, ie on the starboard side for a right-handed propeller. That is the best way of compensating for the paddlewheel effect of a boat with a single fixed prop. The tug should lie far enough back for its prop to have enough clear water all around. You need plenty of fenders between the two boats. The fore spring, from the bow of the tug to the stern cleat of the tow, does the work when going ahead. Bow and stern lines, in this case more like breast ropes, hold the raft together. If the water is smooth, the bow line may be eased whilst under way to leave the fenders only just touching. An additional back spring, from the tug's stern to the tow's bow, is only needed if a lot of manoeuvring and going astern is envisaged; in this case, it will take most of the strain when reversing.

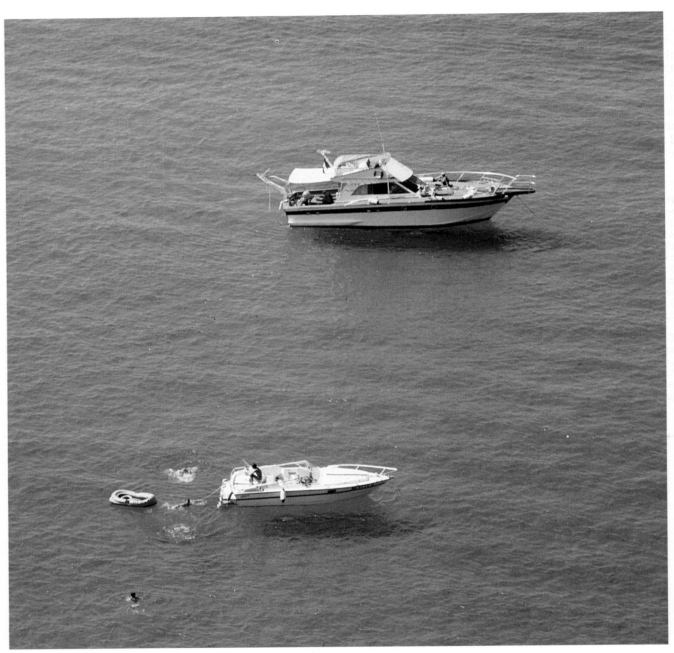

A motor boat provides access to those magical bays inaccessible from the shore, and to picturesque coasts. To be at anchor on a summer's day and enjoying swimming and sunbathing, is a memorable experience.

Anchors and anchoring techniques

Anchors come in various designs and shapes, and sometimes with qualities that are questionable. Only a few have the approval of the institutions concerned with ship safety, such as Lloyds. Proven and preferred for most motor boats are the Danforth and the plough or CQR anchor. The Danforth holds well in mud, sand and clay marl, but has difficulty penetrating an overgrown bottom. The CQR anchor starts to dig in at once, with the pull horizontal along its ploughshare-arm. In sandy and overgrown ground, it holds best of all the designs, except perhaps the old-fashioned Fisherman's anchor. Recently, the Bruce anchor has become popular. Developed originally for oil platforms, its special quality is a high holding power to weight ratio in almost any type of ground. It can, however, be correspondingly difficult to break out. Only in thick weed does it hold less well than the Danforth, because of its shovel-like fluke. If the boat swings a lot about its anchor in a shifting wind or current, the Bruce tends to break out rather easily.

Right: **The most common types of anchor**
1 Bruce anchor. Unless it can be stowed in a suitable fitting at the bow, the Bruce is somewhat awkward to accommodate down below.
2 Plough or CQR anchor. Generally considered a good general purpose anchor with reliable holding power.
3 The Danforth anchor folded flat is easy to stow on board.

Below: Always ready for use: A CQR anchor firmly stowed in the bow roller eliminates any stowage problem and saves work when anchoring. A crossbar or locking pin prevents the anchor from jumping out in a seaway.

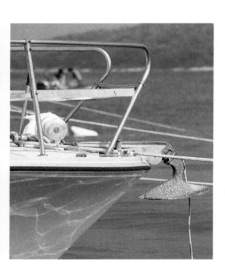

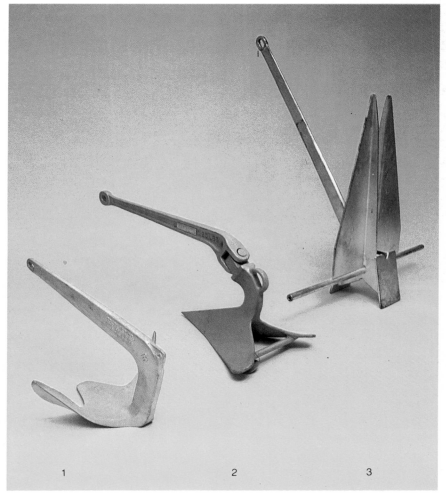

1   2   3

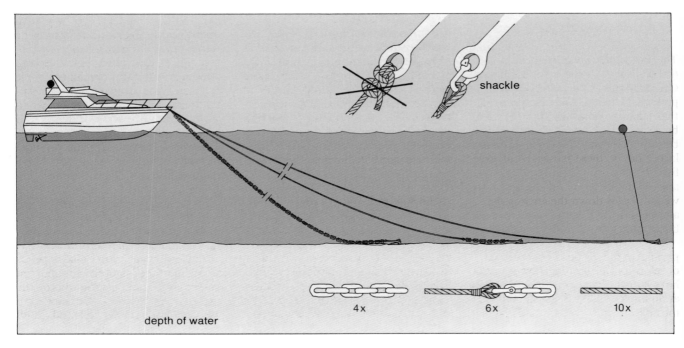

shackle

4 x   6 x   10x

depth of water

How much scope should you give?

Anchoring with chain alone: At least three times the depth of water at high tide.

Anchoring with part rope, part chain: At least four times the depth of water at high tide.

Anchoring with rope alone: At least five times the depth of water at high tide.

These recommendations apply in quiet water. More scope will be needed in strong winds or fast tidal streams.

Though some call it an 'anchor bend', a fisherman's bend should not be used (as often suggested) for bending the cable to the anchor ring. Not only does it not hold well with smooth synthetic cordage, it also reduces the tensile strength of the rope by some 50%. The proper link between anchor and cable is a spliced eye and shackle. An anchor buoy tells us, and others, where our anchor is, and is used to break out the anchor if it becomes jammed in a rock on the seabed. When lying at anchor you should hoist a black ball in daylight and show an all-round white light at night.

Naturally the weight of the anchor is an important factor in its effectiveness, and from that point of view an anchor can't really be heavy enough.

However, the need to handle the anchor sets a natural limit to its weight. The table opposite gives some recommended anchor weights for different sized boats.

Although, according to this table, a second anchor is only recommended for boats of two tonnes weight (displacement) and upwards, even small boats ought to carry a second anchor as a spare.

Weight of boat (tonnes)	Weight of	
	1. anchor (kg)	2. anchor (kg)
0.5	5	—
0.6	5.5	—
0.75	6.5	—
1.0	7.5	—
1.5	8.7	—
2.0	14.0	11
3.0	16.0	11
4.0	17.0	12
5.0	18.0	12
6.0	20.0	14
8.0	23.0	16

Chain or rope?

The longer the anchor chain or rope (cable), the better the anchor holds. On planing craft in particular, rope is preferred. It is handier, much lighter than chain, and by virtue of its high breaking strain and elasticity can even be superior. But if rope is used on larger boats, there has to be at least five metres of chain between the anchor and rope. The chain, by its weight, holds down the anchor shank and helps keep the pull to the anchor horizontal.

Only when the shank is roughly parallel to the sea bed does the anchor develop its full holding power. Tests have shown that, even if the shank is at an angle of only 20° to the bottom, the holding power is halved. The short length of chain prevents the boat giving the cable too much of a jerk, which would raise the shank and might break out the anchor. On rocky ground it helps protect the cable against chafing. The disadvantage of rope as against chain is that it needs a longer scope for the same holding power. You therefore need more room when anchoring because the longer cable substantially increases the swing circle.

There are various reasons for anchoring; perhaps in order to swim and dive off a deserted, idyllic beach. You might anchor to obtain temporary shelter in a bay or estuary, or maybe to wait for sufficient rise of tide to enter a particular harbour or river. You may have to anchor, because night navigation is forbidden on certain inland waterways. You might also have to anchor in an emergency, with engine or steering trouble, to stop the boat from drifting into danger.

If you've got plenty of time and want to anchor for more than a couple of hours, you need to choose your anchorage with care. Ideally, you'll want to tuck into a bay or inlet out of the tide or current and sheltered from the wind. You also need to take account of any forecast or likely changes in wind direction. But lying immediately under a steep cliff, in its apparent lee, is not necessarily advisable. Powerful squalls can come down off the cliff which make the anchorage extremely uncomfortable. The security of an anchorage also depends on the nature of the bottom, and you can find information about this on the relevant charts. Mud and sand give the best holding. Gravel and small

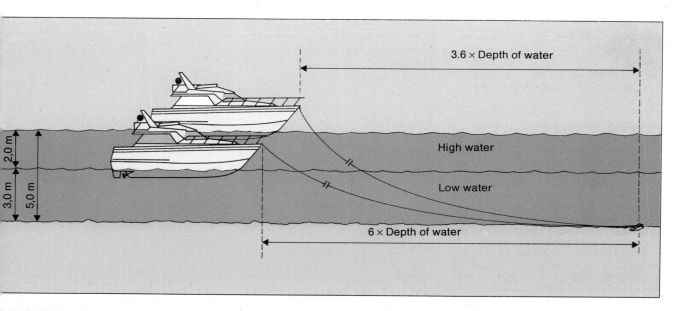

n tidal waters it is necessary to include e depth at high water in your calcula- ons if you anchor at low water and intend to stay that long. If, in this example, there is a 2 metre rise and fall, the rise will reduce the sixfold length of cable to only 3.6 × the depth of water, which may not be enough to keep the anchor shank lying on the bottom.

stones are not exactly ideal but generally cause no problems. A rocky bottom, much overgrown with weed is always risky for anchoring.

Whether on inland or in coastal waters, you must never anchor in a fairway, and you must stay far enough from other boats at anchor to allow everyone swinging room if the wind or the current. should change direction.

A well-known motor boater likes to tell the story of the old sea captain, grown grey sailing the oceans of the world, who was once cruising with him and whom he asked to drop the anchor over the side. The anchor and 30 metres of cable disappeared below the surface never to be seen again – the end had not been secured aboard the boat. This was, in fact, negligence on the part of the owner, since the end of the anchor cable should always be secured in the cable locker or to a cleat or bollard. If the anchor is not stowed permanently at the bow but in a

Anchoring in rocky bays
Neither charts nor echo sounders are completely reliable guides because not every lump of rock is charted, and by the time the echo sounder indicates danger it may already be too late. So you shouldn't chance your arm with such apparently idyllic anchorages unless you can see the bottom clearly. It is often said that you can judge the depth approximately by the colour of the water, but that calls for a lot of experience because various factors such as the sun's position and the nature of the bottom (colour of rocks and weed) play an important part. Very clear water often gives a premature impression of being dangerously shallow. So keep watching the echo sounder when you're feeling your way into such an anchorage.

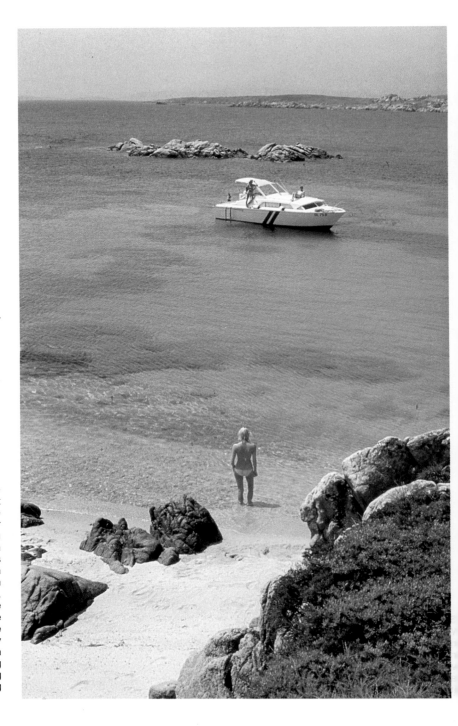

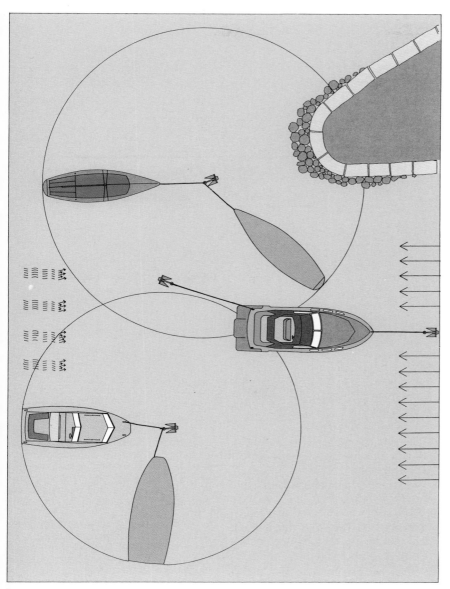

locker, you should fetch it up on deck in good time and run the cable through your hands to check that there are no kinks. You can either coil it down ready to let go or flake it on the foredeck in long loops.

One anchor or two?

Motoring slowing, you round up into wind or current – whichever is the stronger – and go into neutral a little way before your chosen spot. A touch in reverse will bring the boat to a stop and just starting to drift astern, and then you lower the anchor steadily, paying out the cable gradually once the anchor has touched the bottom. If you are lowering the anchor by hand rather than using a winch, never throw all the cable after the anchor; it could drop on top of the anchor, foul it and so prevent it digging in properly. Motor astern very slowly, letting out cable as you go, until you have paid out about three times the depth of water. Then briefly belay the cable, or stop the winch, to jerk the anchor and dig it in securely. Then you can pay out more cable as required. When the boat has reached its final position and the cable is firmly secured, you can briefly nudge astern to check whether the anchor is really holding. If it drags, you have to pay out more cable. If that doesn't help either, there is nothing for it but to pull up the anchor and start again, hoping for better luck next time.

But even an anchor which holds well at first may later – for whatever reason – start dragging. An indication of this is the cable jerking or vibrating, but on a very muddy bottom the cable may behave perfectly normally, as

Swinging about the anchor
With wind or current from one direction, most boats should swing together and not get too close to one another. But if wind and current are in opposition, boats at anchor soon take up different positions. As a rule, a shallow-draught motor yacht will lie predominantly head to wind, while a deep-draught sailing yacht usually swings to the current. Watch out for boats with bow and stern anchors out. They don't join in the swing, but stay more or less in the same place as wind and current change direction.

though the anchor were holding. To establish whether it is indeed holding, you should try to line up two landmarks ashore and watch them for some time to see if their bearing changes. Minor changes usually only mean that the boat is swinging, but if the boat keeps pointing in the same direction while the landmarks move out of line, the anchor is dragging. Modern echo sounders sometimes have an anchor watch facility, but this will only sound if the depth of water changes appreciably.

Strongly gusting and shifting wind places the ground tackle and cleats under enormous strain as the cable alternately pulls taut and falls slack. In these circumstances it can be better to lie two anchors, one ahead and one astern. This is also recommended to reduce your swinging room in a narrow tidal river. You lay the first anchor normally, then drop back and pay out about twice the length of cable required (ie at least *six* times the depth of water). Let this come taut and then drop the second anchor aft. Going ahead very slowly you then haul in half the cable from the first anchor ahead, paying out a corresponding length for the second anchor. It is usually best to secure the end of the second anchor cable forward so that the boat pivots about the two.

To weigh anchor, first drop back to the anchor astern, either by drifting or by motoring astern (in the latter case keeping the line to that anchor taut to prevent it fouling the prop). You then weigh the 'second' anchor and run up to the one ahead. You edge up to it very slowly – simultaneously hauling in the cable hand over hand or using the winch – and then overrun it slightly. Usually the anchor breaks

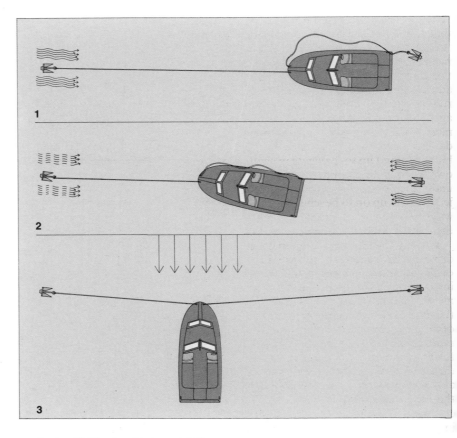

out by itself. You haul it in carefully to stop it banging against the side, rinse it clean and bring it on deck.

Sometimes the anchor is not quite so willing to come up, perhaps because it has got tangled in weed or embedded too deeply in thick mud. Then you belay the cable securely as soon as it is 'up-and-down' and over-run the anchor slowly with the engine, gradually using more throttle as required. If this doesn't work you can try circling the anchor with the cable secured, in order to find a direction of pull on the shank which will enable you to break it free.

Lying to two anchors
1 Drop astern and pay out the bow anchor cable to about twice its required length. Then lower the second anchor aft, paying out plenty of cable and making fast temporarily to the stern cleat.
2 Now haul the boat slowly towards the bow anchor cable again, letting out stern cable as required. In quiet weather you can lie moored bow and stern between the two anchors.
3 In a cross-wind or strong current it is better to take the second anchor forward as well. The boat can then lie easily to both anchors, one of which will be holding securely whatever the direction of wind or current. Swinging room is much reduced.

Driving a jet

A few years ago people were saying that the hydrojet was going to bring the jet age to boating. This development has not quite lived up to expectations, and yet it seems to have so many advantages. There is no propeller or rudder to be damaged by going aground or which can injure swimmers. With a jet you can, without damage, run over any obstacle the hull will stand up to, navigate in shallows (a good 10 centimetres of water under the bottom are enough for the jet) and run up on to beaches and slipways without any problems. Why then, has it not become more popular?

Driving a jet is very different from driving a propeller-driven boat. First of all you notice an unusual indicating instrument on the fascia – the vacuum meter. To be able to draw in water for the reaction jet, the impeller must first of all generate a partial vacuum. The more marked this is, the more powerful the 'suction' and the greater the thrust. A drop in the vacuum inevitably means a drop in performance, so the importance of this instrument is comparable to that of the rev counter in propeller boats.

Since going astern is achieved entirely by the deflector, there is no reversing gear. Whether going ahead or astern, the impeller shaft keeps turning in the same direction. This allows you to do something which is impossible with any propeller boat – to go from full ahead to full astern without touching the throttle. The boat stops almost on the spot; enveloped by a cloud of spray and with a little leap in the air if it's a lightweight. Of course the opportunity for such an impressive display will normally be pretty rare, but it's nice to know you can do it. Also, using the water jet the boat can be turned literally in its own

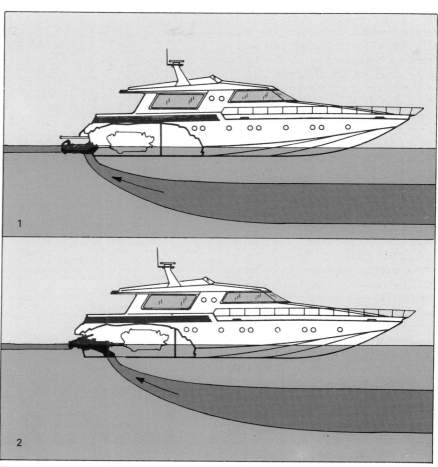

There are two types of jet installation – outboard or inboard

1 Outboard: The complete unit is suspended from the transom. This means that the impeller draws in the water to be accelerated from outside the boat, directly via a grating in the unit. Mounting and maintenance are simple, but the rigid unit, projecting horizontally a long way, forms a long lever arm. The forces acting on it have to be absorbed by the transom and the coupling flange, which can produce structural problems.

2 Inboard: The drive unit is substantially inside the hull and draws its water through a grating in the bottom. If the boat leaps over the waves, the impeller starts swallowing air a lot sooner than with an outboard unit. This can mean added wear on engine and transmission.

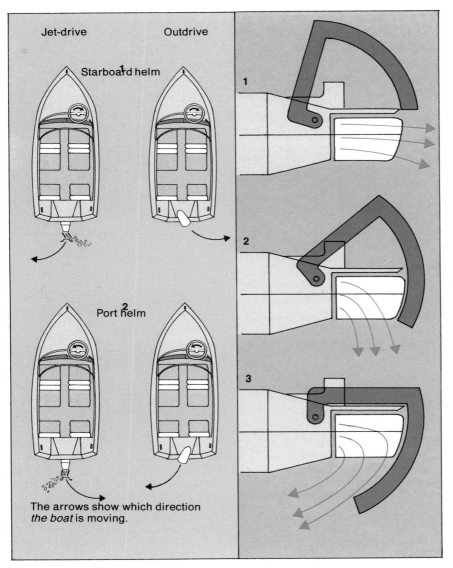

Jet-drive   Outdrive

Starboard helm

Port helm

The arrows show which direction
the boat is moving.

Left: **Thrust reversal with the deflector**
(reversing scoop):
1 Going ahead
2 Neutral (idling). Port or starboard
rudder applied with the deflector in this
position makes the boat rotate about its
axis without moving either ahead or
astern.
3 Reversing.

length – on the spot. This is an impressive characteristic, and water-jet enthusiasts never fail to give it due emphasis. Of course they sometimes overlook the fact that yachts with twin props can do that too.

Driving a jet-propelled boat calls for a totally new technique. Pressure on the helm is almost imperceptible and at displacement speeds steering a straight course can be difficult until you get the feel of things. Only at higher speeds does the course stability approach that of propeller boats. Going astern calls for a lot of rethinking. A prop-drive angled to the right pulls the boat's after end to the right too; turning the steering wheel the same way in a jet-driven boat produces exactly the opposite effect, ie movement to the left. And, of course, the other way with a left turn.

There is also something else new for prop-boat skippers to learn about: a third control to operate. In addition to the steering wheel and throttle you have the 'joystick' for the deflector. All these tricks can of course be learnt, and once you have really got the hang of this 'Wurlitzer' you may even succeed in making your boat move practically sideways. And the somewhat eccentric characteristics when manoeuvring astern are something you soon get used to.

Above left: **Handling jet-drive boats in
reverse**
There are two types of 'bucket' deflector which can be used with an inboard jet drive. When the deflector is attached to the nozzle, steering is just like steering an outdrive. However, when the deflector is attached to the stern of the boat and is separate from the nozzle, steering in reverse is 'back to front' – when you turn the wheel to the right the jet boat turns astern to the left (1) and vice versa (2).

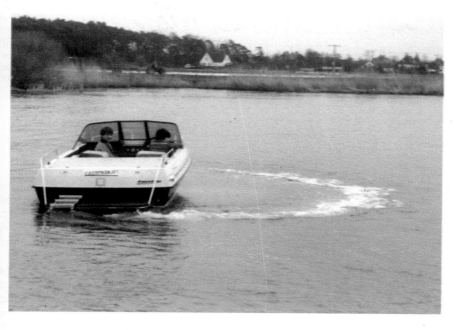

Driving a jet in rough water requires great skill if the boat starts to leap in the air. Anyone who cares for his engine has to juggle constantly with the throttle because the drive pump – the impeller – starts to race much more easily than a propeller when it leaves the water. For this reason some hydrojet engines have rev limiters, which automatically prevent the engine overspeeding in those circumstances. One jet-drive builder has re-located the intake duct and impeller actually within the propulsion unit, aft of the transom, so the drive is less prone to be starved of water.

Jet-driven boats need to be driven fast. Even at about 80% of maximum revs – which is normally a fast economical speed for a prop-drive – speed may be only about 50% of maximum. Many of them can only be made to plane by increasing the engine revs to near the maximum rated speed. Jet drives are therefore relatively thirsty. It also follows that they are unsuitable for displacement craft. A prop-driven boat at half revs reaches something like half speed; a jet-driven boat reaches, at best, quarter speed. The explanation for this lies in the amount of 'squirt' which different engine revs can generate. The nozzle diameter is designed for the maximum revs of the engine, so if the impeller is only moving half that amount of water, the exit nozzle no longer runs at full pressure. Instead of the jet squirting out of the nozzle full of energy under high pressure, producing bags of thrust, it dribbles feebly into the sea and the boat only creeps along. If sea conditions force you to throttle back from full power the efficiency of a jet-drive drops quickly. If you enjoy driving jet boats you have to accept a relatively heavy fuel consumption, particularly since the overall efficiency is no more than 75% of that of a propeller.

Seaweed can be a problem for small jet-drives. The protective grating at the inlet of the suction duct can become choked, and if you're unlucky the boat may even have to be lifted out of the water to clear the blockage. To solve this problem, the Italian jet builder Castoldi fits a folding rake for clearing any seaweed remotely. But neither this nor various other improvements seem able to increase the popularity of jet-drives amongst the boating fraternity. The major American outdrive manufacturer, who in the initial phase of jet euphoria started developing jet-drives, is now mainly restricting its designs to specialist rescue craft and certain military applications.

However, the hydro-jet has managed to retain a toehold in the field of sporting craft, because it is available for engines up to 1200 hp for twin and triple installations suitable for driving large high-speed offshore racers. The technical problems of transmission which arise with high horsepower engines are largely eliminated by using jet drives. Economy, of course, is no longer a consideration – only maximum speed by any means and at any price.

129

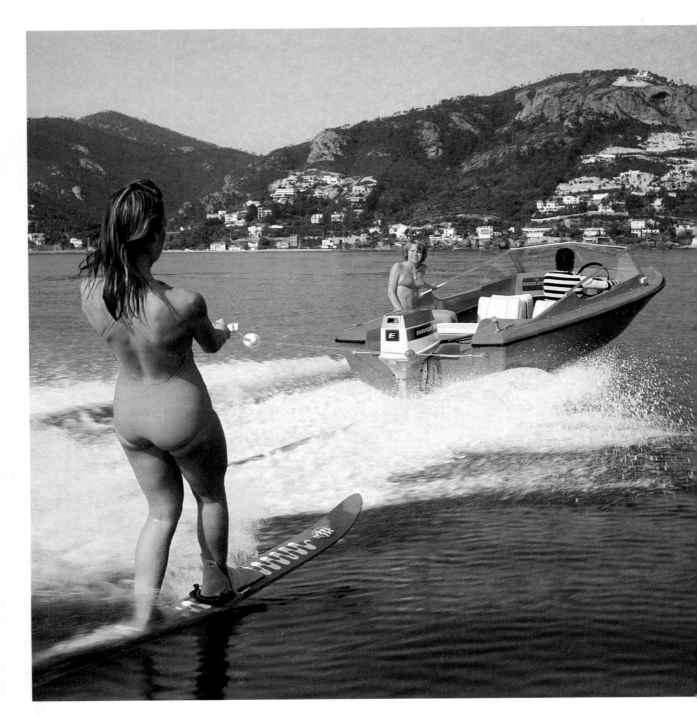

Water skiing

There is a band of enthusiasts who say that it takes water skiing to make motor boating a real pleasure. For these people, a motor boat is merely a means for towing them over the water at high speed on a couple of boards. Water skiing is certainly an exhilarating experience, and you get a tremendous sensation of speed from hissing over the surface of a calm blue sea. It takes a while to learn the knack of getting up though, and beginners should resign themselves to a long succession of false starts before they finally manage to take off on a decent run.

As a towing boat, almost any properly powered planing craft is suitable, although it rather depends on what sort of demands the skier makes. There is, of course, a lower limit in terms of power and speed. The boat should get up to at least 14 or 15 knots with four people on board because the power needed to tow a water skier is roughly the same as two passengers require. This relationship holds true for speeds up to about 25 knots. There must always be a co-driver in the boat to keep a constant eye on the skier. Just a rear view mirror for the driver is not enough, though it is strongly recommended. For inflatables and very light outboard engined boats,

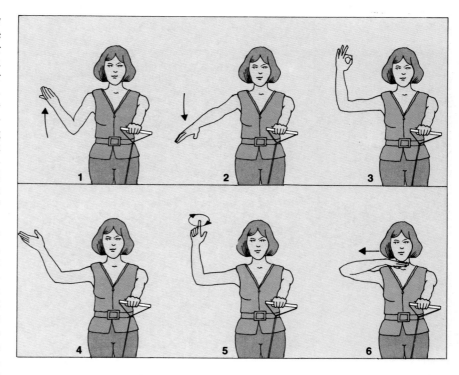

When water-skiing, communication by voice is scarcely possible because of the noise made by boat and skis, so skier and observer have to communicate using an unambiguous sign language. There may be some regional variations in the hand signals, but they will be understood nevertheless.
1 Palm (or thumb) upwards: faster.

2 Palm (or thumb) downwards: slower.
3 AOK. Speed just right.
4 Turn (to the right in the example).
5 Index finger (or whole hand) rotating: turn round; run over the same stretch of water again.
6 'Throat-cutting' gesture: finish, back to the shore.

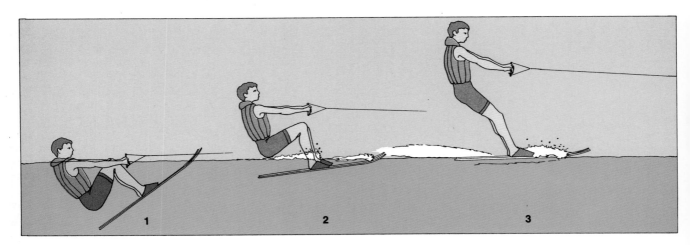

Starting from the water

1   In water about chest deep, go into a crouching position. Stretch out the arms horizontally at shoulder level and press against the knees which are together, with feet and skis about a hand's breadth apart. The skis should just stick out of the water, angled about 40° to the horizontal. The tow-rope runs between the ski tips. Your seat should be about a hand's length above the back ends of the skis. You wait for the pull to start.

2   The boat starts towing. Arms stretched, knees close together, stay crouched (don't try to stand up) and with your back straight just let the boat pull you up. Don't look down, look along the tow-line, at the stern of the boat, otherwise you're liable to become 'top-heavy' and lose your balance. In this position the skis should, by themselves, become progressively flatter and finally start to plane properly, the skier only just skimming the water with his seat. Now stand

upright using your ankles and knees, not pulling yourself up on the tow-bar. Back and arms should remain straight while you stand up, bottom pulled in . . .

3   Done it! You have achieved the final skiing posture. Keep the hands roughly level with your bottom ribs and at no time straighten out the   knees entirely — always keep them slightly bent and flex them in response to the waves.

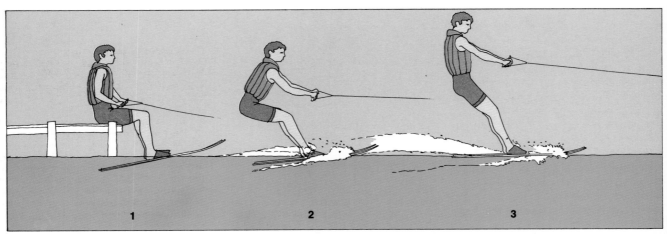

The dry start

Sometimes you can start from a landing-stage or directly from a deck or bathing platform. The dry start differs from the start from the water in one basic respect

— the arms are initially held at an angle (1) to absorb the initial tug of the tow-rope gradually. You sit with skis submerged as far as the bindings. Arms and legs slightly bent, you allow yourself to

be pulled from the stage without pushing-off (2). You balance during this phase by slightly bending/stretching your arms. Once the skis are planing, take up the skiing posture (3).

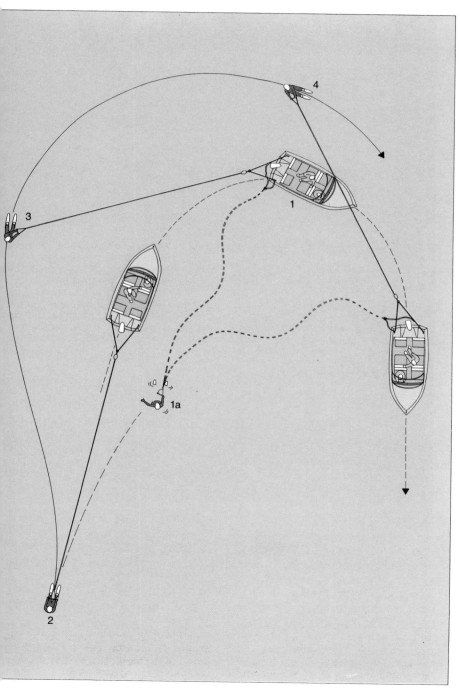

25 hp (18 kW) is about the minimum power needed for normal water-skiing. The more demanding monoski needs 40 hp (29 kW).

Naturally the weight of the skier has to be taken into account. Lower power requirements, as promised by some sports boat brochures, are usually over optimistic. The speed at which the experts really start enjoying themselves is 18–20 knots, but to achieve this requires more horse-power. In some respects though, the more horsepower you have for skiing the better. The greater the power, the more quickly the skier is lifted out of the water. He or she can then concentrate properly on skiing instead of first having to plough through the water a long way until the skis have enough lift. A boat with insufficient power can't maintain a steady speed as the load on the tow line varies; it will slow down and speed up again as the skier

The technique of turning
1 The boat makes a sharp turn. Wrong: the skier is initially pulled into the turn but then the tow-rope develops slack and he becomes submerged so far that he has to break off (1a).
2 Correct: the skier initially sheers off (in this case to the left) out of the wake, in such a way as to cross the stern wave at an angle of about 45°. He does so by applying a little more heel pressure to the left ski; the ski at once starts to turn in that direction. Reducing the heel pressure and loading both skis equally again, automatically reverts him to running straight.
3 When you get here the game starts again, this time with pressure from the right heel, for a turn to the right.
4 And the same again. This way you continuously maintain tension in the rope and stay up on the skis.

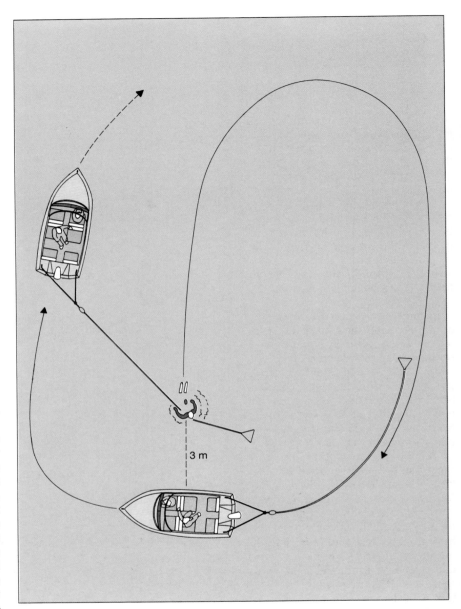

Falling and starting again from the water:
If your skier has fallen – which will
happen pretty frequently to a novice –
you turn back in a gradual circle. The
tow-rope is pulled along until the boat is
behind and at least 3 metres away from
the swimmer. Now turn hard-over and
continue slowly roughly at right angles.
The tow-rope cuts the corner and is
pulled directly past the skier in the water
until he can grab hold of the bar. Then
stop the engine and start again.

3 m

meets waves. The resulting jerky tension in the tow line can easily cause a beginner to fall.

Differences in boat and hull design produce significant differences in wake and stern waves. What you want in a towing boat is as flat a wake as possible, which means not a lot of 'V' in the aft part of the hull, but nevertheless good turn stability. You really do need the latter to prevent the stern from being dragged off course by the side swings of the skier. Furthermore, the wake of the ideal towing boat should not spread too far and, at the centre, should be stirred up as little as possible by rudder and prop. The crests of the waves generated should not be steep but gently rounded. Some of these requirements are barely reconcilable, so you usually end up with a satisfactory compromise.

The type of engine and how it is installed also has a part to play in the type of stern wave you have. The engines of boats used professionally for towing water skiers are sited amidships and drive a fixed shaft. The midship centre of gravity results in a very well balanced trim; the fixed shaft and rudder create a smoother central wake than the shafts of outboards and outdrives. An outboard is preferable to

an outdrive, producing a 'ski-friendly' wake so long as the hull is right. For that reason, anyone still a bit insecure on skis will prefer a boat with an outboard.

Boats specially designed for towing have a 'mast' for the tow line, situated forward of the stern to make turning easier. Otherwise, the tow load should be split between two eyebolts in the transom using a bridle, with a running sheave on it for the tow rope. A little

further back you should have a float, to stop the bridle from fouling the prop when the load is off it.

You're not allowed to water ski just anywhere. It is totally forbidden on canals and in harbour areas. On rivers, skiing is usually only permitted on certain designated stretches, sometimes marked off by buoys. Skiing may also be restricted to certain times or days of the week. One more thing to remember – a boat towing a water skier must give way *absolutely* to all other boats. You must also keep a safe distance, bearing in mind the swing of the tow-rope, from beaches, swimmers, river banks and other sports boats.

The standard tow-line length is 23 metres, but for small boats with outboards this is usually shortened to 18 metres. Although swinging out on this scope is great fun, a skier should always stay within the wake of the towing boat when overtaking or meeting other boats.

Beginners who succeed in staying on the skis after the start will first try to follow the relatively smooth wake of the towing boat, keeping a straight course as far as possible. But you can't just go on skiing in a straight line. Sooner or later you'll have to make a turn. The driver should at first make his turns very wide and gentle, using only a little helm. This allows the skier to remain in the wake. The skier should shift his or her weight to the 'inside' ski with the boat. If the boat is forced to make a tight turn, the novice skier will be in trouble. The tension in the tow rope will suddenly drop and he'll probably lose speed and sink. In order to keep the tow rope continuously under tension and keep up his speed the skier must make a wider turn than the towing boat.

Falling into the water is no disgrace for a skier. If you realise that a fall is inevitable, let go the towing handle at once. This will ensure you a 'soft landing' and you'll sink gradually into the water. The thing to avoid is hanging on to the handle desperately, because you are then likely to hit the water pretty hard and may be dragged along.

The time will come to return to the beach. Nothing could be simpler. The

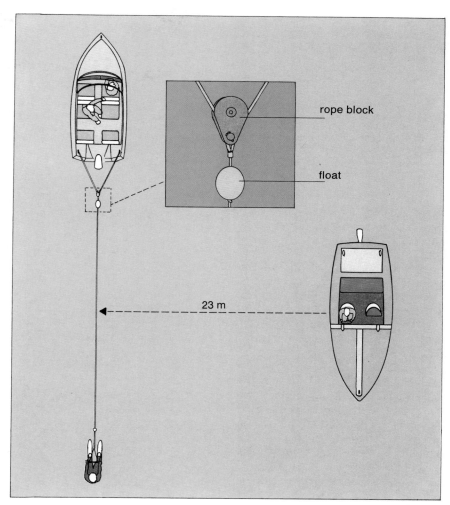

rope block

float

23 m

driver approaches the shore and reduces speed; the skier gradually sinks further into the water, finally lets go the tow handle, takes off the skis, and swims the last few yards to the beach. The 'dry feet' landing is of course more spectacular; the boat approaches the beach or jetty at normal towing speed and then turns away, while the skier lets go of the handle and, with the remaining momentum, carries straight on to end

A boat with a water skier must give way to all other boats, keeping at a safe distance in the process – usually at least a tow-rope length.

up close to the beach or jetty with a flourish. This requires accurate judgement and is not always possible, because in many places the shore may only be approached slowly and at right angles.

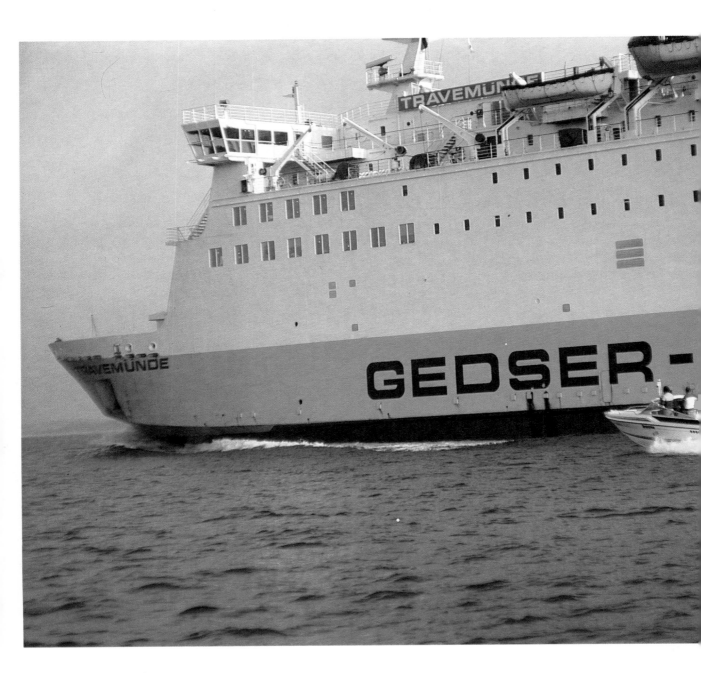

An easily manoeuvrable motor boat should always keep out of the way of large ships. This is both sound seamanship and common sense.

Traffic regulations –
who gives way to whom?

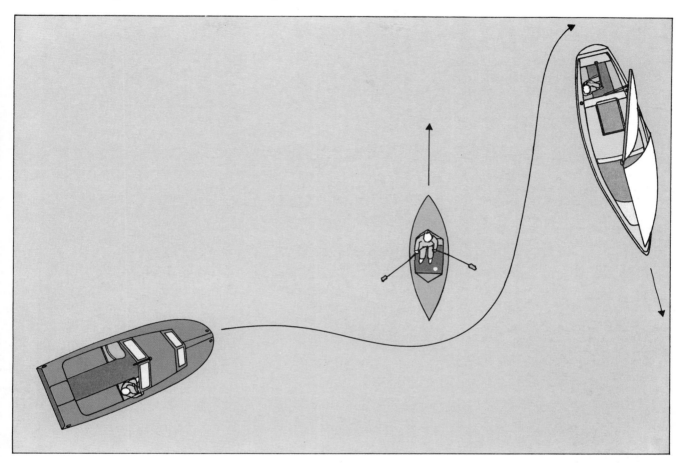

Apart from the vastness of oceans, which a motor boat crew scarcely ever experiences, there is almost nowhere on the water where you are completely alone. On the contrary, near harbours and in rivers there can be a considerable crush. Your freedom of the seas may end all too quickly when you are faced with the looming steel bulk of a ferry, a container ship or a supertanker. Just as on the roads, there are rules for responding to other traffic to avoid chaos developing.

Seaborne traffic is controlled by an internationally agreed set of 'Rules of the Road' – the 'International Regulations for Preventing Collisions at Sea'. These regulations lay down the courses of action to take when you meet other vessels in various circumstances, both at sea and in more restricted waters. They also cover the use of lights at night and sound signals in poor visibility.

Giving way to rowing and sailing boats: Unless the latter are using their auxiliary engine, a motor boat is always the give way vessel, regardless of which side they approach from. Similarly, motor boats always give way to rowing boats. The only exceptions to this general rule are when a rowing or sailing boat is overtaking a motor boat, in which case the overtaking boat always keeps clear.

As far as traffic regulations are concerned, there is one basic respect in which inland waterways and port areas differ from the open sea, and that is that recreational craft must give way to all merchant vessels. At sea, on the other hand, motor boats and yachts enjoy, in theory at least, equal status with merchant ships.

However, small boats – and this includes most motor yachts – should always try to avoid a situation in which they meet a large vessel at close quarters. When such an encounter does take place, the rules lay down clearly what action should be taken and by whom. But bear in mind that,

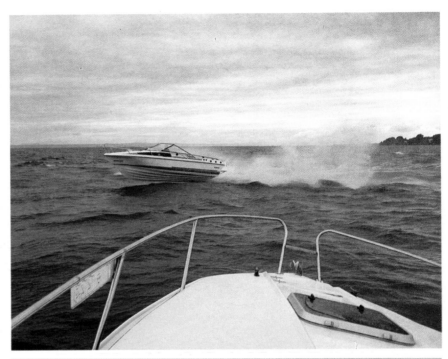

Motor boats meeting: the boat coming from starboard and seeing the other to port has the right of way.

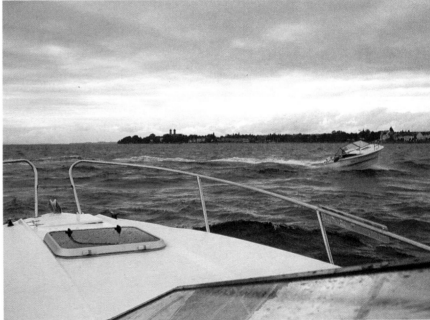

If two boats on opposing courses approach one another so as to pass at a safe distance, neither need alter course. They can then (as here) pass starboard-to-starboard. This rule also applies at sea between merchant ships.

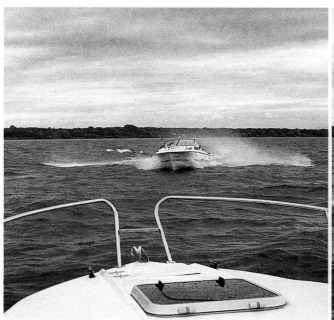

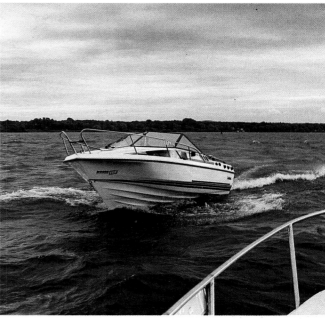

Two boats closing from opposite directions so that there is a risk of collision must both alter course to starboard. They then pass port-to-port.

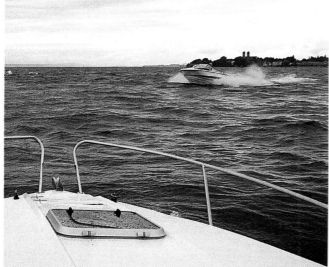

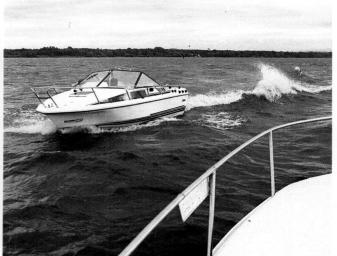

If you're approaching from port and see the other boat to starboard, you have to give way. Either stop the engine until the other is past or, better still, alter course to starboard to let the other pass to port and then turn under his stern.

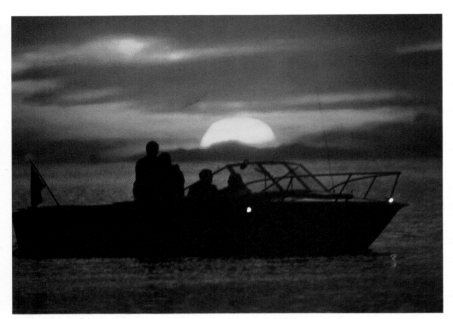

Optical illusion? From the silhouette of the boat, what is facing you here is her starboard side, so you have the right of way. However, the green side light looks white to the eye in this case, creating a misleading impression. Always be careful when interpreting small boat lights. They are often not bright enough and are sometimes angled incorrectly.

When two motor vessels are meeting head-on, or nearly head-on, both should alter course to starboard and pass port side to port side. Motor boats always give way to yachts under sail or to rowing boats.

If you are overtaking any other boat or vessel you have to give way. You may pass on the left or the right, depending on the traffic situation and what seems most advantageous to you. If you are turning from a secondary channel into a main fairway (rather like a major road) you must not impede the traffic in the main fairway, eg by forcing another ship to make an emergency turn.

In daylight, with good visibility, everything is relatively easy. It is a good deal more difficult in darkness, when all you have to go on are other ships' steaming and navigation lights which appear here and there in the gloom. Working out the right course of action is by no means easy and requires some experience to interpret and assess the direction of traffic and its distance away. Newcomers to boating are well advised not to start off by involving themselves in night navigation, especially where there are traffic lanes used by merchant shipping. Instead, novices should seize every opportunity to take part as crew in night passages made by experienced skippers.

whilst it is an easy manner for a motor boat to alter course, slow down or come to a dead stop, this is certainly not true of large merchant ships.

The other important point to realise is that, whilst a motor boat helmsman can easily see a large merchant ship or ferry in clear weather, the officer of the watch on the bridge of that ship cannot necessarily see a small motor boat bobbing about in time to take avoiding action.

Any craft whose duty it is under the Rules to give way must alter course positively and in good time. What you mustn't do is make several small alterations of course in succession. The other vessel might not notice these at all and could, as a result, react wrongly or start to take avoiding action himself. A distinct alteration of course of 90° where courses are crossing clarifies the situation beyond doubt.

The Rules lay down that when two motor vessels (which includes two motor boats or a merchant ship and a motor boat) are crossing, so as to avoid risk of collision, the one which has the other on her own starboard side shall keep out of the way and shall, whenever possible, avoid crossing ahead of the other. The vessel which has right of way should maintain her course and speed to avoid confusing the situation.

At night, all you can see of other boats or ships are their navigation lights, so you have to work out from these who has to give way. For that you need not only sharp eyes but also a certain amount of experience. Knowing the arcs of visibility of the various navigation lights is important for deciding in which direction particular ships are heading.

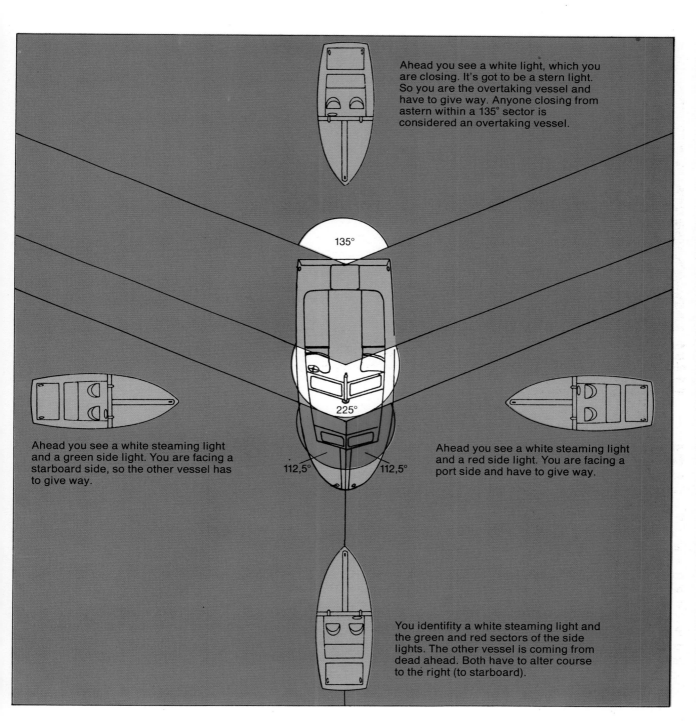

Ahead you see a white light, which you
are closing. It's got to be a stern light.
So you are the overtaking vessel and
have to give way. Anyone closing from
astern within a 135° sector is
considered an overtaking vessel.

135°

225°

Ahead you see a white steaming light
and a green side light. You are facing a
starboard side, so the other vessel has
to give way.

112,5°   112,5°

Ahead you see a white steaming light
and a red side light. You are facing a
port side and have to give way.

You identifity a white steaming light and
the green and red sectors of the side
lights. The other vessel is coming from
dead ahead. Both have to alter course
to the right (to starboard).

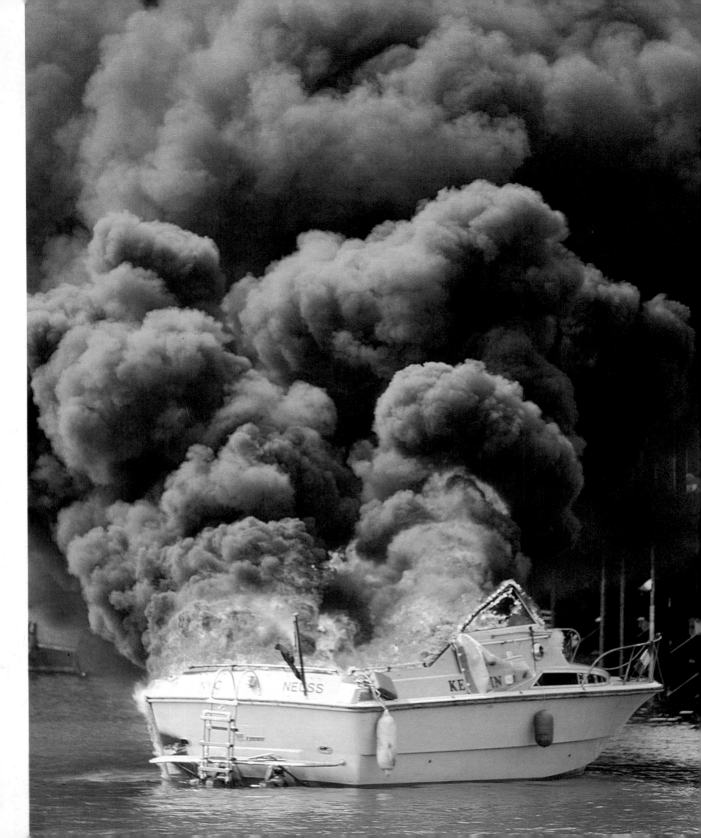

Fire on board – what to do?

The possibility of a fire on board a motor boat can never be totally excluded, but you can aim to take careful precautionary measures. So here, for a start, are six pieces of advice worth following:

- Always see to it that the bilge and all drip trays underneath engines and cookers are clean and dry.
- In normal weather, try to ensure the effective through-ventilation of all compartments. Never shut off the ventilation to fuel tank, battery and engine compartments.
- Try to check regularly your gas installation and engine fuel systems, and all associated containers, fittings, pipelines and hose clips.
- Maintain all electrical wiring and equipment in good condition. Check all connectors frequently and tighten any that are loose. Secure any cables that come loose and repair damaged insulation at once. Cables whose insulation has become brittle, or defective switches, should be renewed without delay.
- An engine that misfires, particularly a petrol engine which is flashing back into the carburettor, should be shut down at once to avoid the risk of a carburettor fire. Look for the cause before trying to restart the engine.
- Have all fire extinguishers serviced regularly and make sure you have plenty of them.

The engine, even if it is petrol, is not necessarily the principal source of danger. Life in the galley is relatively risky because cookers are a frequent cause of fires. Gas cookers are obviously dangerous if there are any gas leaks, but badly-maintained 'safe' paraffin cookers can also be a risk. If not preheated sufficiently, they can spit out an alarming jet of flame which has often been the cause of curtains or deckhead cladding catching fire. Strongly heated fat ignited by the cooker flame licking over the pan edge can also cause a jet of flame to shoot upwards. Even cookers using pressurised meths can, on occasion, produce unexpected fireworks. LPG (butane, propane) can turn into a bomb on board if carelessly handled. If containers or connections leak, the gas, being heavier than air, can trickle down into the bilge and accumulate, lurking there until an accidental spark sends you sky high. So painstaking attention has to be given to the proper installation of all gas bottles.

The recommended place to keep

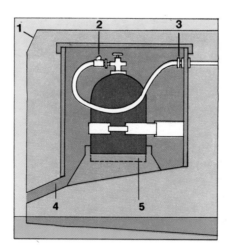

A safe gas bottle installation
1 A box separated by bulkheads from the other spaces.
2 Safety pressure regulator.
3 Screwed bulkhead gland.
4 Above-water drain for any escaping gas.
5 Secure mounting for the bottle.

A two-bottle installation additionally has a bottle safety valve and a manual changeover valve.

gas bottles is on deck, outside the living quarters, in a well vented locker. To allow any gas that might escape to run away, a downward-sloping drain pipe must lead from the lowest point of the locker directly over the side. The only equipment that should be used with gas are cookers, heaters, refrigerators or ovens with proper fail-safe cut-outs. These automatically interrupt the gas supply if, for instance, a draught blows out the flame. Another valuable safety device is a built-in electronic gas sniffer, which sets off an alarm if there is even a slight escape of gas.

There are various types of fire extinguisher, each being suitable for certain types of fire. But which kind should you have and how many do you need if what you hope will never happen should happen? Let us have a look at what can be extinguished with what. Halon (dichlorofluoromethane) has substantially replaced the previously popular CO_2 extinguisher systems in engine compartments. Halon is much more effective than carbon dioxide, and the best medium also for manual extinguishers. It arrests the combustion process by smothering it at once; the fire goes out instantly. Since even a concentration of only 4% by volume of Halon is enough to achieve extinction, it is not even necessary to aim accurately as you have to with a powder extinguisher. Being non-conducting, Halons are eminently suitable for putting out electric installation fires. Being gases, they penetrate even to the hidden centre of a fire, and they leave behind neither pollutants nor residues. You can even turn the extinguisher briefly on people, eg to extinguish burning clothing. The snag about this apparently ideal extinguishing medium is that, in contact with glowing metal and in

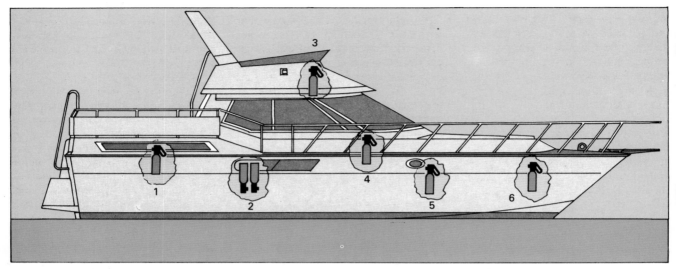

Strategic positions for mounting Halon or powder extinguishers

1 A 2-kg extinguisher in the after cabin, with a second in the aft bathroom if a gas water heater is fitted.

2 A permanent Halon extinguisher system in the engine compartment, with a second possibly in the tank space. Capacity depends on the size of the engine compartment.

3 A 2-kg extinguisher at the helm position on the flybridge.

4 A 6-kg extinguisher at the helm position in the saloon.

5 A 6-kg extinguisher for the galley and main cabin.

6 A 2-kg extinguisher in the forward cabin.

conjunction with open flames, it generates small quantities of toxic gas. For this reason all enclosed spaces – which in practice means all cabins – should be cleared of people within a minute of a Halon being used.

The popular dry powder extinguisher is an all-purpose extinguisher for all types of fire. The non-poisonous powder melts when it makes contact with fire and covers the area with a glassy substance. The fire is smothered but the material extinguished is not cooled. It continues to generate vapour, so you have to follow up with water as soon as possible. Gas-water extinguishers are suitable only for incandescent fires (class A). They deal with these most effectively because of their powerful cooling effect and penetration, but in most cases you could

		Fires involving solids principally of an organic nature, which normally form an incandescent mass. eg wood, paper, straw, coal, textiles, car tyres	Fires involving liquids or melting substances eg petrol, oil, greases, varnish, resins, wax, tar, ether, alcohol, synthetics	Fires involving gases eg methane, propane, hydrogen, acetylene, mains gas	Fires involving metals eg lithium, sodium, potassium, aluminium and their alloys
Suitable					
Suitability limited					
Different types of fire and suitable extinguishers					
Dry powder extinguisher					
Halon extinguisher					
Gas-water extinguisher					

achieve the same result with a couple of buckets of freely available water.

All fire extinguishers must receive proper maintenance regularly – at least every two years.

Some recommended accessories for the smaller extinguishers are an additional hose and spray-nozzle to allow access to the awkward corners when fighting a fire, and an interruptor lever so that you can operate the extinguisher in bursts. The larger extinguishers have these facilities as standard. All extinguishers must be mounted so as to be immediately accessible in the event of a fire, without the operator having to waste time fighting with a jammed or rusted catch. If mounting and catch are not made of non-rusting material, they should have a coating of plastic as corrosion protection.

The number of extinguishers required depends on the size of the boat and on the flammability of the equipment fitted. For a boat with an outboard, one 2 kg dry powder extinguisher within reach of the driver may be quite sufficient. On larger boats there should be several extinguishers strategically placed throughout the accommodation. Engine compartments on larger boats are often fitted with a remote controlled extinguisher system. It is no use mounting manual extinguishers inside the engine compartment – if a fire starts here, nobody will be able to reach them. For boats of more than about 150 hp (110 kW), a fixed Halon extinguisher system is suitable for the engine compartment. This can be combined with an automatically-triggering temperature sensor or smoke detector, but must also be operable remotely from the helm position(s).

You should have at least two extinguishers in or near the galley, particularly if there is a gas oven, gas cooker or gas fridge. If there is a hot water geyser in the lavatory/shower room, you should have an extinguisher there too. Every cabin should have at least one 2 kg extinguisher. If there is no fixed extinguisher system in the engine compartment, there should be manual extinguishers outside by the access.

Fighting a fire

Minor fires, such as those liable to flare up in the galley, are most quickly dealt with by smothering with a blanket of fireproof foil. These blankets are available in various sizes. Carburettor fires are also best tackled with a smothering blanket, or you can pack a wet woollen blanket around the carburettor instead. As well as trying to put a fire out you also have to try to cut off its oxygen supply. If possible close doors, windows and scuttles and try to turn the boat relative to the wind so that the flames are not driven back over the craft but rather away from it. Then stop the engine, because motion through the water and the engine itself convey large amounts of oxygen into the boat via the ventilation system. If cables are burning, switch off the power if you can before fighting the fire. Use the main battery switch if you can reach it. Once the fire is out, you have to try to establish in which fuse circuit it started. Then you can isolate this separately and restore the main power.

To be able to fight a fire effectively you must get as close to it as possible. Don't waste an extinguisher until you can use it effectively because you'll be surprised how quickly they run out. A 2 kg extinguisher will be finished in about 8 seconds and a 6 kg one in 10 to 12 seconds. That's precious little time, so you can see why you need plenty of extinguishers aboard a boat. Don't direct the jet at the flame itself but at the actual parts that are burning. If possible, approach the heart of the fire bent double or crawling, because low down there will be less flames, less smoke, better visibility and the most breathable air. When using a manual extinguisher in the engine compartment, open the hatch or engine cover only just enough to be able to insert the spray nozzle. As you lift the cover, turn your head away as far as possible so that if a jet of flame does shoot out it won't hit you in the face. If you have to operate below decks, first thoroughly drench your clothes and tie a wet cloth around nose and mouth. Come out at intervals to get some fresh air, and try not to breathe in smoke and fumes in the cabin.

If plastic fittings or the plastic hull itself are already burning and a lot of smoke has been generated, don't under any circumstances go below again. Highly poisonous vapours are generated which in a matter of seconds can cause unconsciousness and long-term damage to health.

Foam-filled cushions are best thrown overboard after the flames have been extinguished as they carry on smouldering for ages. Special care is required with internal cladding; not only can the fire spread behind it unnoticed, but after you have (apparently) put the fire out, it may continue to smoulder out of sight and suddenly break out again. If you have been extinguishing or following up with water, don't forget to start the bilge pump afterwards if it's still working. Otherwise, the excess water will have to be pumped out by hand.

Engine breakdowns and fault finding

A well and regularly maintained boat engine – whether outboard or inboard – is, generally speaking, pretty reliable in operation. If it does become more trouble prone than a car engine, the explanation probably lies in the harsh environmental conditions afloat (the boat engine's worst enemy is corrosion) and because it is not being run often enough. A boat engine needs more tender loving care than a car engine, so your most important ally is the operating manual. Everyone should study this carefully before starting the engine for the first time. Don't wait until you are bobbing up and down in the middle of a fairway with a stopped engine before desperately leafing through the manual for the first time. A full workshop manual can also be useful, although engine manufacturers are usually reluctant, or may refuse altogether, to hand these out. They fear, with some justification, that owners would fiddle too much with their engines.

There are many different types of boat engine – outboard, petrol inboard, diesel inboard – and a breakdown can be caused by a whole range of factors. For that reason we can include here only general advice applicable to most engines, and some of those tricks that must be mastered by everyone who drives a motor boat. The checklists are intended to point you in the right direction when trying to find the fault, before you start to search the operating manual.

Fault-finding: Outboard engines

Engine vibrates heavily	Oil pressure low (4-stroke)	Engine overheats	Engine stops when gear is engaged	Boat does not attain normal speed	Engine does not attain full rated revs	Speed decreases in spite of rev increases	Uneven running or spark cut-out	Rough idling	Engine starts and then stops	Engine won't start	No tension in hand starter cord	Starter does not turn engine	Possible cause	Remedy
												●	Battery terminals loose or corroded	Remove terminals, clean with a wire brush or emery cloth, replace and tighten well
												●	Battery too low	Start engine with a 2nd battery and jump leads, or remove and charge battery
												●	Starter defective	Remove starter for repair or take complete engine to workshop
											●		Hook or spring of starter defective; starter cord parted	Many engines have a recess in the flywheel for starting with an emergency cord. In some cases this requires removal of a cover or the hand starter (see operating manual)
										●			Fuel pump defective	Remove pump and exchange for a new one. Repair, by engineer, is only possible with the right spare parts
									●	●			Fuel hose not connected	Connect hose and prime with fuel using the squeeze pump connected
				●	●		●	●	●	●			Fuel hose kinked	Apply only gradual bends to the fuel hoses. Take care not to stand cans or the tank on the hose
				●	●		●	●	●	●			Fuel filter dirty	Depending on the type, (gauze or paper cartridge) fuel filters must be cleaned or renewed at least once per season (see operating manual)
				●	●		●	●	●	●			Water in fuel system	Drain carburettor, pump and filter, pipelines and tank. Clean and then blow through with compressed air. Refill tank with clean fuel
										●			No spark	Modern ignition systems can't be checked reliably without special tools. Unless it is just a question of cleaning or replacing spark plugs, the engine has to go to workshop for repair
		●		●	●		●	●	●	●			Plugs dirty or defective	Unscrew plugs and clean with a wire brush. Set electrodes as per maker's instructions (see operating manual). Plugs with damaged/burnt electrodes must be changed
										●			Leads wrongly connected	Connect leads in right order (see operating manual)
									●	●			Engine flooded	Unscrew plugs, replace in plug sockets and short leads to engine block. This prevents damage to ignition system. Open throttle fully and turn engine over Replace plugs, fit leads and start engine

Fault-finding: Outboard engines

Engine vibrates heavily	Oil pressure low (4-stroke)	Engine overheats	Engine stops when gear is engaged	Boat does not attain normal speed	Engine does not attain full rated revs	Speed decreases in spite of rev increases	Uneven running or spark cut-out	Rough idling	Engine starts and then stops	Engine won't start	No tension in hand starter cord	Starter does not turn engine	Possible cause	Remedy
				●	●			●	●	●			Carburettor badly adjusted	Have the carburettor adjusted by a recommended engineer
		●		●	●		●	●					Too much oil in fuel mixture	Drain fuel system and refill with correct mixture (see operating manual)
		●		●	●		●	●	●				Plugs with wrong heat value	Remove plugs and replace with ones of the right heat value (see operating manual)
		●		●	●		●	●	●	●			Weak and irregular spark	Ignition systems can't be checked reliably without special tools. Engine has to go to workshop for repair
		●		●	●		●	●					Spark too far advanced	Spark timing can't be adjusted properly without special tools. Another job for experts
				●	●		●	●					Spark too far retarded	Spark timing can't be adjusted properly without special tools. Another job for experts
									●	●			Tank vent closed	Always check that tank vent is open before starting
						●							Shear-pin sheared	Unscrew prop nut, extract broken pin and replace with new. Always carry spare shear pins
						●							Prop safety clutch defective	Can usually only be repaired by a listed engineer
						●							Propeller lost	Every boat should carry a spare propeller, shearing pins, split pins and a prop nut
				●	●								Propeller with wrong pitch	Only careful trial runs with a rev counter will indicate when you have a correctly pitched propeller. Max revs attained must be closed to the rated revs given by the engine manufacturer (see operating manual)
●				●	●								Prop damaged	Damaged props must be changed as soon as possible, otherwise transmission bearings will be damaged
				●	●								Transom not high enough	The engine shaft length must match the boat's transom height (about 38 cm for short shaft and 51 cm for long shaft engines)
										●		●	Ignition lock defective	Replace lock. In an emergency the starter solenoid can usually be bridged with a cable or a screwdriver
		●		●	●								Cooling system choked	May be due to salt crystals, weed or sand. Cleaning should always be carried out by an expert
		●		●	●								Water pump defective	A defective water pump always means some dismantling of the engine's underwater portion. A job for experts
				●									Transom too high	The engine shaft length must match the boat's transom height (38 cm for short shaft and 51 cm for long shaft engines)
●			●	●	●								Fouled propeller	Fishing lines, ropes and plastic bags must be cut away with a knife. In stubborn cases this may mean taking off the prop
			●										Transmission jammed	A leak allowing water into the transmission or loss of oil, are the usual causes of inadequate lubrication. If an oil change does not cure the problem, the engine has to go to experts for repair
	●												Engine is short of oil	Replenish oil as instructed by manufacturers, just up to maximum-level mark (see operating manual)
	●												Oil pump defective	Here only experts can help
	●												Oil quality and viscosity wrong	Drain engine oil and refill with fresh complying with manufacturer's instructions (see operating manual)
●													Engine loose on transom	The engine-mounting bolts and T-screws must be checked for tightness at regular intervals. Any that are loose, tighten at once
●													Engine block mounts loose	At least once per season the components of the flexible engine block mounts must be checked carefully, nuts and bolts tightened, defective mounts renewed
		●		●	●		●	●	●				Air leakage in fuel system	Check fuel system pipes and connections. Replace porous pipes and defective connections

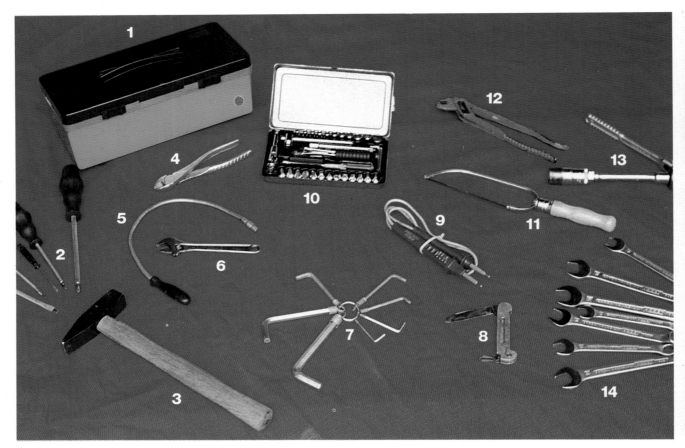

The tool kit

1 Tool box
2 Screwdrivers for slotted and Phillips screws
3 Hammer
4 Side cutting pliers
5 Bar magnet
6 Adjustable spanner
7 Set of keys for Allen set screws
8 Knife
9 Voltage detector with polarity indicator
10 Box of socket spanners
11 Hacksaw
12 Special pliers for water pump
13 Plug spanner
14 Ring/open-ended spanners

Engines sometimes break down a long way from any engineers or workshops, so you ought to have a good tool kit on board. The more frequent emergency repairs include changing V-belts, plugs, propellers on outboard motors, and the impeller for the water cooling. If a water pump impeller runs dry because of a closed seacock or a plastic bag over the inlet, it is usually damaged so badly that it has to be renewed. A defective cooling water thermostat is not repairable on board unless you carry a spare. Otherwise, it has to be removed from the circuit until you get to the next port-of-call, to protect the engine against overheating. Cleaning the sea water filter is one of the simpler tasks. Dirt or water in the fuel is a frequent cause of engine breakdowns, and you need to check the fuel filters and water separators regularly.

Steel toolboxes are an irritating source of rust, so use only plastic boxes. You should always carry a suitably-sized plug spanner, long-nosed pliers for removing the pump impeller, side cutting pliers, a

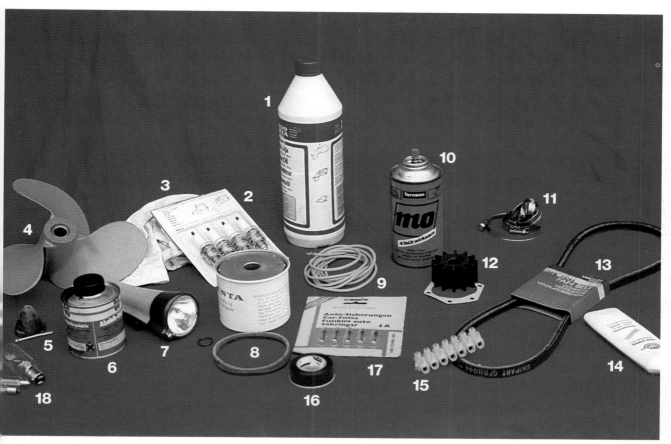

medium-sized hammer and a good set of screwdrivers, both for slotted and Phillips screws. To check on the electrics you will find a decent multi-meter – well worth its weight – plus a small electrical screwdriver. Knife and hacksaw are indispensable, especially for cutting away any rope or other debris from an outboard or outdrive. You will also need special tools for changing props, and a good quality set of open ended and ring spanners (metric or imperial, depending on your engine).

A basic outfit of spare parts comprises alternator drive belt, fuel filters, water pump impeller and cover gasket, prop with parts for holding and locking it, fuses for all the circuits on board, engine oil and oil filters. Petrol engines, in addition, need as many plugs as there are cylinders, a spare coil and a set of points. Absolutely necessary are insulating tape, stainless steel and copper wire, 'chocolate block' electrical connectors, a reel of two-core electrical cable, sealant, water-resistant grease, rust solvent spray for terminals, and spare bulbs for navigation lights, panel instrument lights, navigating equipment and cabin lights.

1 Engine oil
2 Plugs
3 Cleaning cloth
4 Prop
5 Prop nut with split pin
6 Sealant
7 Pocket torch
8 Fuel filter with sealing rings
9 Spare flex
10 Rust solvent spray
11 Stainless steel 'Jubilee' clips for hose connections
12 Impeller with seal
13 V-belt
14 Water resistant grease
15 Strip connectors
16 Insulating tape
17 Fuses
18 Spare light bulbs

Spark plugs

Spark plugs may seem very ordinary components, but they perform, for petrol engines, one of the most vital functions. If neglected, they can produce major breakdowns. Plugs are exposed to extreme working conditions, but are nevertheless always expected to ensure reliable running of the engine – whether when cold-starting or at maximum output. They have to tolerate voltages which can exceed 30,000 V and combustion pressures of up to 50 bar. In the course of a single working cycle, a plug may be exposed to changing temperatures ranging from 120°C to 3000°C. For every engine manufacturers prescribe plugs with a specific heat value. If you want trouble-free running from an engine, especially from an outboard, you simple must use these and no other plugs. They are precisely attuned to the engine's compression, running speed, cooling and carburettor setting. Depending on the engine load, all plugs should normally operate in a temperature range somewhere between 400°C and 850°C. The lower limit is called the limit of free combustion, and this must be attained rapidly after starting. If the plug is too cold, soot deposits will build up on the electrodes and insulating collar, and the ignition energy is greatly reduced. If fouling becomes excessive, the spark may disappear altogether. However, the cause of the soot formation may not necessarily be a wrong type of plug; it may also be due to a rich mixture setting, a defective automatic choke or a dirty air filter. If, on the other hand, a spark plug gets too hot, the fuel-air mixture may be ignited prematurely and cause lasting damage to the engine.

Combustion residues on the plug change its appearance and, from observing these changes, you can deduce, fairly reliably, various causes of trouble. You can only draw such conclusions from a spark plug after the engine has been running on load for about ten minutes. If, by then, the insulating collar is not a whitish to

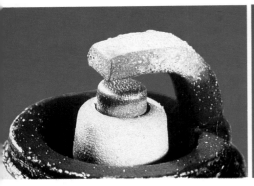

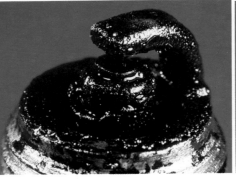

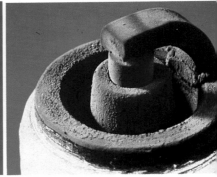

Assessing engine performance from the spark plugs
1   Colour of end of insulator ranging from whitish grey through yellowish grey to fawn. The heat value is correct and the engine in good order.

2   End of insulator, electrodes and plug body are coated with oily soot or oily coke.
Possible causes:
Too much oil in combustion chamber, oil level too high, badly worn piston rings, cylinder and valve guides. With 2-strokes, too much oil in the mixture.
Effects:
Intermittent ignition; cold starting difficult.
Remedy:
Have engine overhauled, correct fuel-oil mixture, fit new plugs.

3   End of insulator, electrodes and plug body are coated with velvety, dull black soot.
Possible causes:
Wrong mixture setting (carburettor, injectors), mixture too rich, air filter very dirty, automatic choke defective or choke left out too long, plug running too cold/heat value too high.
Effects:
Intermittent ignition; cold starting difficult.
Remedy:
Correct mixture and cold start settings check choke; check air filter and clean if necessary.

yellowish grey, but instead you see the first signs of deposits, either the plug has the wrong heat value or there is something wrong with the engine.

To make sure of a reliable spark, the plugs should be taken out and checked regularly. If they are oiled-up or have an oily-carbon deposit, they must be cleaned, preferably with a wire brush. If there is heavy fouling, don't waste a lot of time trying to get them clean, just fit new ones.

Before screwing in a cleaned or new plug, check whether the electrode gap is correct as laid down by the manufacturer, using a set of feeler gauges. The gap can be opened carefully with a knife blade or tapped closer with a spanner. The appropriate feeler gauge should just slide through the gap. Plugs for high power capacitor ignition systems usually have an angular electrode in place of the curved bar. They can be cleaned just like conventional plugs, but you cannot adjust the gap. They must be renewed at once if the central electrode looks pointed and no longer projects above the angular electrode.

Finally, remember that plugs are subject to normal wear and tear. The interval for changing them will be indicated by the engine manufacturer, and it's a false economy to try to squeeze more life out of them than this.

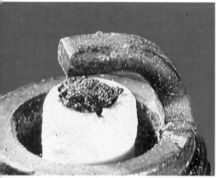 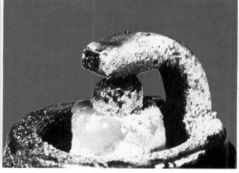 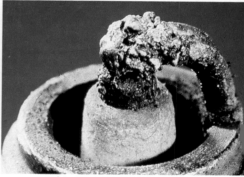

4 Central electrode melted away; insulator tip spongily softened or bubbly.
Possible causes:
Excessive thermal loading due to pre-ignition, eg ignition too far advanced; combustion residues in combustion chamber; defective valves; defective distributor; fuel quality low; heat value of spark plug too low.
Effects:
Intermittent ignition, loss of power (damage to engine).
Remedy:
Have engine, ignition system and mixture preparation checked; fit new plugs.

5 Insulator end has thick yellowish-brown or greenish glaze locally.
Possible causes:
Lead-rich fuel additive. The glaze will often form when the engine is loaded heavily after a lengthy run at part load.
Effects:
The coating becomes electrically conductive and makes ignition intermittent.
Remedy:
New plugs; cleaning is useless.

6 Electrodes cauliflower-like in appearance. Possibly deposition of extraneous material.
Possible causes:
Excessive thermal loading due to pre-ignition, eg ignition too far advanced; combustion residues in combustion chamber; defective valves; defective distributor; fuel quality low.
Effects:
Substantial power loss and risk of serious engine damage.
Remedy:
Have engine, ignition system and mixture preparation checked; fit new plugs.

Fault-finding: Inboard engines

Charging indicator lamp remains on	Oil pressure low	Engine vibrates heavily	Engine overheats	Fuel consumption excessive	Engine stops when gear is engaged	Speed decreases in spite of rev increases	Boat does not attain normal speed	Engine does not attain full rated revs	Uneven running or spark cut-out	Rough idling	Engine starts and then stops	Engine won't start	Starter does not turn engine	Possible cause	Remedy
													●	Main switch not on	Switch on main switch
													●	Gear lever not in neutral	Some manufacturers fit a safety switch in the transmission, which interrupts the starter circuit if the engine is in gear. Before starting always check lever is in neutral
													●	Engine main fuse defective	Change fuse (see operating manual). If it happens again, have the system checked by a marine electrician
													●	Ignition lock defective	Change lock. In an emergency the starter solenoid can usually be bridged with a cable or a screwdriver
													●	Battery flat	Start with a second battery and jump leads, or remove and charge battery
													●	Battery terminals loose or corroded	Remove terminals, clean with a wire brush or emery cloth, replace and tighten well
													●	Starter defective	Remove starter for workshop repair
												●		Heater plugs defective (diesel)	Heater plugs must be checked by an engineer at regular intervals. Defective plugs must be changed
											●	●		Fuel cock shut	Always make sure that fuel cocks are all open before starting
							●	●	●	●	●	●		Fuel link kinked	Fuel lines should have gradual bends. Do not set anything (cans, gear) down on fuel hoses
											●	●		Fuel supply pump defective	Remove pump and exchange for a new one. Repair by an engineer is possible with the right spare parts
							●	●	●	●	●	●		Injection pump defective	Repairs to and adjustments of injection pumps may only be carried out by experts
							●	●	●	●	●	●		Fuel filter dirty	Depending on the type (gauze or paper cartridge), fuel filters must be cleaned or renewed at least once per season (see operating manual)
							●	●	●	●	●	●		Water in fuel	Water separators, fitted separately or as sumps on tanks, must be drained and cleaned at regular intervals. If water gets into the fuel system, the whole system (tank, pipelines, filter, supply and injection pump, injectors or carburettor) must be drained and cleaned. Refill tank with clean fuel. Diesel engine fuel systems must be bled free of air as instructed by the manufacturer (see operating manual)
							●	●	●	●	●	●		Air in fuel system	Check fuel system pipelines and connections. Renew any leaky, porous or defective pipes, or defective connections. Diesel fuel systems must be bled free of air after any work involving removal of a fuel component (eg a filter) or drainage of the fuel (see operating manual)
				●			●	●	●		●	●		Weak irregular spark (petrol engines)	Ignition system components can't be checked or repaired reliably without special tools. The engine must be taken to listed engineer
				●			●	●	●	●	●	●		Plugs dirty or defective (petrol engines)	Unscrew plugs and clean with a wire brush. Set electrodes as per maker's instructions (see operating manual). Plugs with damaged/burnt electrodes must be changed
				●			●	●	●		●	●		Injection nozzles	Nozzles must be checked by experts at regular intervals (see operating manual)
							●	●	●	●		●		Leads wrongly connected (petrol engines)	Connect leads in right order (see operating manual)
												●		Engine flooded (petrol engines)	Unscrew plugs, replace in plug sockets and short leads to engine block. This prevents damage to ignition system. Open throttle fully and turn engine over. Replace plugs, fit leads and start engine
		●					●	●	●	●	●			Carburettor badly adjusted (petrol engines)	Have carburettor adjusted by a recommended engineer
			●	●			●	●	●	●				Plugs with wrong heat value (petrol engines)	Remove plugs and replace with ones of the right heat value (see operating manual)
			●	●			●	●	●	●	●	●		Distributor defective (petrol engines)	Ignition system components can't be checked or repaired reliably without special tools. Engine must be serviced by an engineer
				●			●	●	●	●	●	●		Contacts defective/ gap wrong (petrol engine)	Renew contact points and set the correct gap using feeler gauges (see operating manual for gap tolerance)

Fault-finding: Inboard engines

Charging indicator lamp remains on	Oil pressure low	Engine vibrates heavily	Engine overheats	Fuel consumption excessive	Engine stops when gear is engaged	Speed decreases in spite of rev increases	Boat does not attain normal speed	Engine does not attain full rated revs	Uneven running or spark cut-out	Rough idling	Engine starts and then stops	Engine won't start	Starter does not turn engine	Possible cause	Remedy
							●	●	●	●	●	●		Moisture in/on ignition system (petrol engines)	Spray parts of system (plug leads and connectors, distributor cover) with water displacing fluid
			●	●			●	●	●	●	●	●		Ignition timing too advanced or retarded	Ignition timing can't be adjusted properly without special tools. Engine must be serviced by an engineer
				●			●	●	●	●	●	●		Air filter (flame trap) dirty	Depending on the type (gauze, oil bath, paper cartridge), air filters must be cleaned or renewed at regular intervals
							●	●						Turbo charger defective	Only specialists can carry out repairs to turbo chargers
							●	●						Propeller with wrong dimensions	Commissioning the boat must include determination of the 'right' propeller, by making trial runs with a rev counter. Maximum revs then attained must be close to the rated revs given by the engine manufacturer (see operating manual)
		●					●	●						Propeller damaged	Damaged props must be changed as soon as possible, otherwise shaft and transmission bearings will suffer excessive wear
		●												Prop shaft bent	Repairs to a fixed shaft or outdrive can only be carried out by experts
			●				●	●						Cooling water inlet seacock shut	Always open cooling water inlet seacock before starting engine
			●				●	●						Sea water filter dirty	Close inlet seacock, open filter, remove and clean gauze
			●				●	●						Shortage of cooling water	Replenish coolant as per manufacturer's instructions (in emergency use clean tap water)
			●				●	●						Cooling water thermostat defective	Exchange thermostat for a new one (see operating manual)
			●				●	●						Cooling water pump defective	A damaged impeller must be changed. Remove dump cover and extract impeller using two screwdrivers or water pump pliers
			●				●	●						Cooling water system choked	Cause can be salt crystals, sand or seaweed. Cleaning system, including heat exchange and oil cooler, should always be carried out by experts
		●			●		●	●						Fouled propeller	In the case of boats with outdrives, fishing line, rope and plastic bags can be cut away with a knife. The prop may have to be taken off. Fixed-shaft boats have to be dried out, slipped, lifted out of the water, or else you need the services of a diver
					●									Transmission, outdrive or shaft jammed	Repairs to outdrive, transmission or fixed shaft should only be carried out by experts
	●		●											Oil shortage	Check engine for oil leaks. Replenish oil to max. mark as per manufacturer's instructions (see operating manual)
	●													Wrong oil quality/viscosity	Drain or pump out oil. Replenish with fresh as per manufacturer's instructions. Change filter (see operating manual)
	●													Oil pump defective	Only experts can help here
	●													Oil filter choked	Replace choked filter by a new one (see operating manual)
		●												Engine mounts defective or loose	At least once per season check all components of the flexible engine mounts, tighten nuts and bolts, renew defective mounts at once
		●												Engine alignment incorrect	Transmission output and prop shaft must not be offset. Alignment of engine and prop shaft can't be checked or corrected without special tools. A job for experts
●			●											V-belt defective or slack	V-belts must be checked and re-tensioned at regular intervals. A slack belt slides on the pulleys, which means that the alternator or cooling water circulating pump operate at reduced output. A properly tensioned belt can be depressed by hand about 5 to 8 mm between pulleys. A belt gone brittle must be exchanged at once
						●								Prop safety clutch defective (outdrives)	Must be repaired by a recommended engineer
			●				●	●						Charge air cooler defective	Only experts can help here

Knots, bends and hitches

It has happened more than once that someone has seen their precious boat, thought to be carefully tied up, floating away into open water. The explanation is often that a self-invented knot, 'safe as houses', was used to make fast the boat's painter, and this knot silently and discreetly just let go. At the other extreme you have the complicated masterpieces which contract to such an extent that the only way they can be undone is with a sharp knife.

The only reliable knots are proper sailor's knots, which have evolved over centuries to be simple to tie, secure and easy to cast off. Motor boaters, and indeed most seamen, only need to know the half dozen most common knots – and what they are used for – to be able to cope with almost any eventuality in their boating careers. However, you have to be able to tie these basic knots quickly and under adverse conditions, per-haps in the dark while hanging upside down over the bow trying to reach an elusive mooring buoy.

Let's take a look at these important basic knots:

The **clove hitch** is for making fast dinghy painters to mooring bars, the rungs of ladders, or stanchions. It is also most commonly used for securing fenders to guardrails.

A round turn and two half hitches is the somewhat awkward name for a secure and quick-to-make knot for fastening a warp or dinghy painter to a ring or crossbar. The great value of this knot is that it can be cast off easily under strain.

The **reef knot** is used for joining two light ropes of the same thickness and material. The knot has to be symmetrical, ie the bare ends must come away from the bight on the same side, otherwise the knot will come undone at once. It is also used for securing lashings using light line.

The single and double **sheet bend** are used to join two ropes together, especially if they are of differing thickness and/or material. If stiff, brittle synthetic rope is involved, the double sheet bend is much to be preferred.

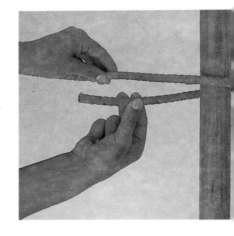

The clove hitch: take the line around the bar or ring like this (called 'taking half a round turn'), ...

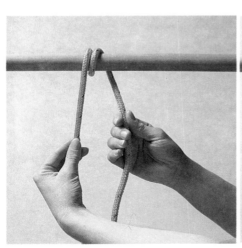

Round turn and two half hitches: take the line twice around the bar like this ...

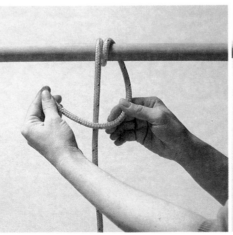

bring the end round in front of the standing part ...

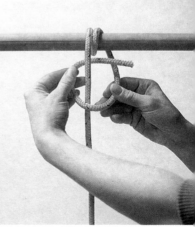

then behind and forward through the loop. ...

154

Even for ropes of the same thickness, a double sheet bend is much better than a reef knot if the ropes are very slippery.

Probably the most commonly used knot is the **bowline**. With this you can make a non-slipping eye of whatever size you like. It is used for making fast to posts, bollards or even rings, although an important disadvantage of the bowline is that it cannot be cast off easily under strain. You can use two interlocked bowlines for joining two heavy warps together, perhaps to make a long tow-line.

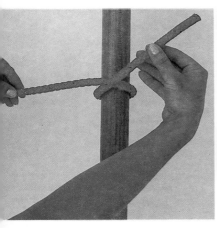

n bring the end up over the standing rt . . .

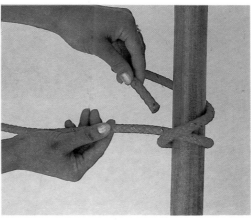

round the bar or ring again . . .

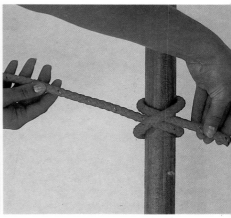

and through under itself where it crosses the standing part and haul taut. The clove hitch is made.

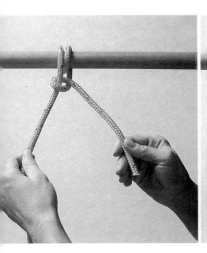

at's what one half hitch looks like. w do the same again: . . .

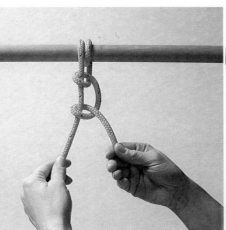

round in front, behind and through the loop . . .

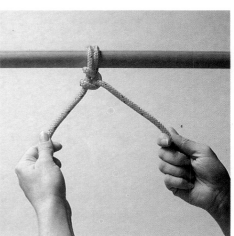

and haul taut. A secure knot, easy to cast off under strain.

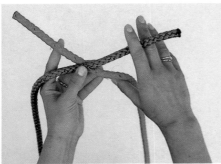

The reef knot: cross the two ends over; hold one (green) between the fingers of the right hand, lead the standing part of the other (red) over the thumb. . . .

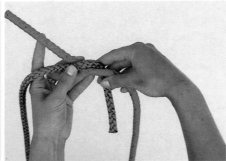

A twist of the right hand to the right . . .

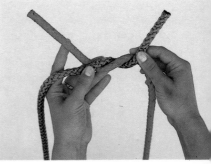

and the two ends are twisted together. The left hand has remained inactive. . . .

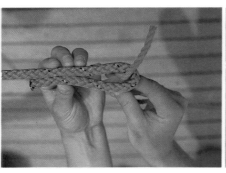

The sheet bend: make a bight (loop) with the end of the thicker line and take the end of the thinner line through . . .

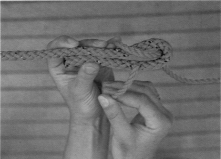

then round the two parts of the bight, nearer the thicker bare end . . .

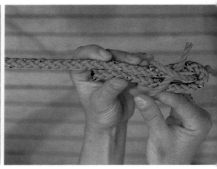

and back over this and through under itself. . . .

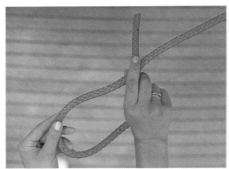

The bowline: take the end in the right hand, parallel to the index finger, and place the thumb underneath the standing part . . .

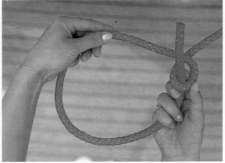

twist the right hand to the right (back of the hand downwards). The end or the rope and finger now project through the small loop so formed . . .

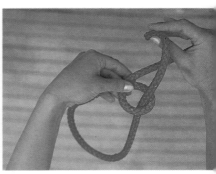

grip that loop between finger and thumb of the left to fix it, take the end with the right . . .

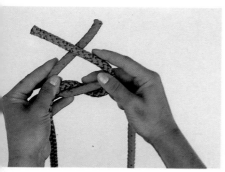

Now the two ends are crossed again, green over red . . .

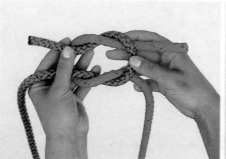

the red then taken around and through under the green, so making two interlocked bights which engage and nip one another. . . .

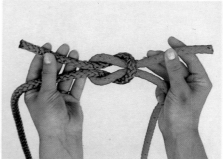

Haul taut and the knot is finished. Remember – left over right, then right over left (or vice versa).

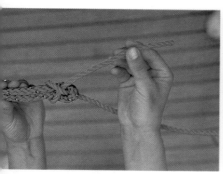

Haul taut and you have made a single sheet bend. . . .

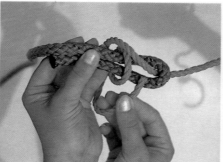

To make a double one, take the thin end round the two parts of the bight again, nearer the head . . .

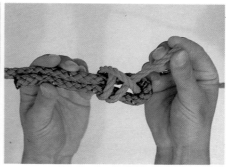

and push it through under itself a second time before hauling taut.

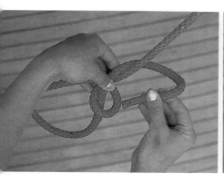

pass it round behind the standing part from the left . . .

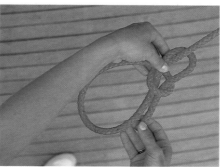

and go back through the eye, then haul taut. With very slippery cordage, . . .

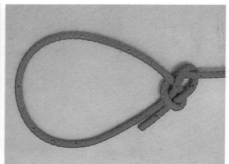

have at least a hand's breadth of bare end projecting from the eye. The large loop so made cannot slip even under extreme loads.

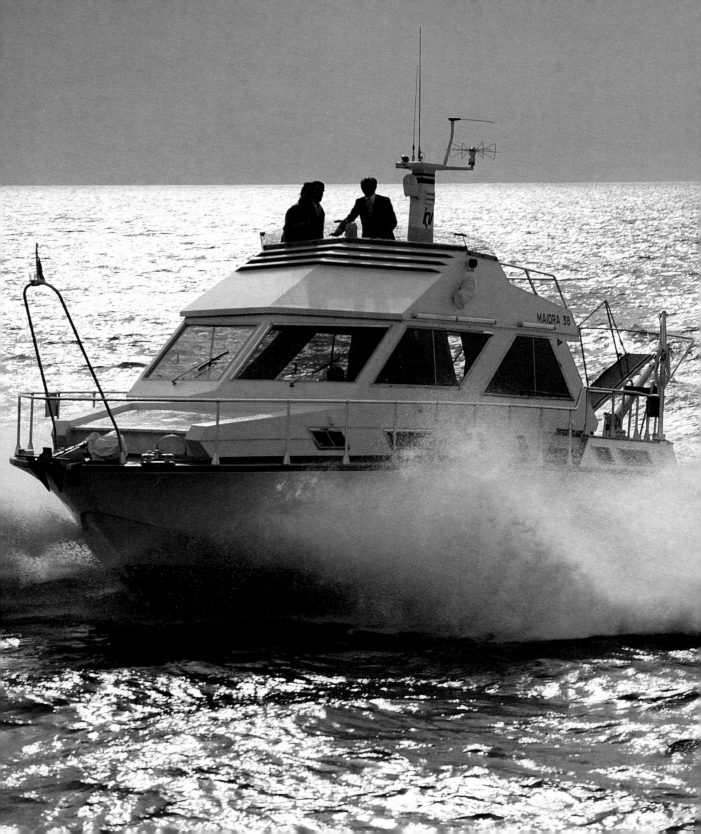

Index